MW00465605

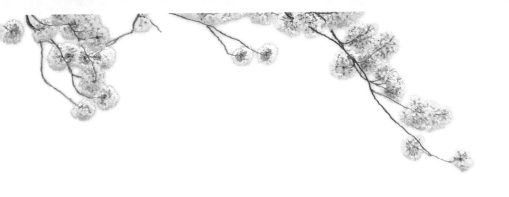

"Reiki produces good health, happiness and security"

Dr. Mikao Usui
Founder of Reiki Natural Healing

2015 TRA
conference
mg 8 —

A loha Reiki Sista,

Enjoy my stories!

R xo R xo,

Shalandra

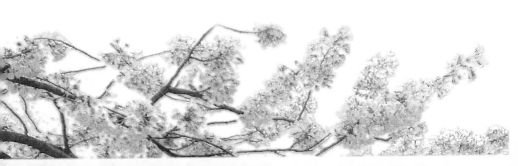

"Best book about Reiki we have ever found. In this highly recommended, easy to read book, Shalandra has not only captured, but faithy conveyed to paper the very essence of living Reiki. She is living proof of the wholeness and joy to be found in choosing to live Reiki."

Gloria and Graham Richardson
Reiki Masters
Western Australia

"The *Eat, Pray, Love* of Reiki. Very inspirational book and a wonderful way to either reconnect or be introduced to the Reiki Energy."

Joanna Wheeler
Sales Executive
Kauai, Hawaii

"This is a beautiful introduction to how Reiki can be in one's life. Shalandra truly lives a life of Reiki, and, is dedicated to sharing Reiki with others. In her book she shares what that means for her. This book is a key part of my personal library, and I heartily recommend it."

Greg Goodson
Reiki Master
Red Bluff, California

"The book was wonderful - very informative and full of insights about Reiki. It would be quite a selling point to someone who is just getting interested in the program."

Jim Miller
Second Degree Reiki Practitioner
Hot Springs Village, Arkansas

"I have read *Living a Life of Reiki* over and over and still get more from it each time I pick it up. I use something I have taken from this book each day to either put me back on track, or stay on track, or just reassure myself I'm on track. And now I am wanting to purchase copies for my students."

Robyn Mckechnie
Reiki Master
Western Australia

"I truly have enjoyed this book. It has given me the kick I needed to remember how important it is to use my Reiki to live a healthy life. I am filled with gratitude for Shalandra and all that she does for the health of so many."

Carol Them
Second Degree Reiki Practitioner
Hendersonville, North Carolina

"Shalandra Abbey takes us through her intimate journey with Reiki with beauty and grace. She leaves you feeling as if you are one of her best friends. Her work is full of heart, healing and real but heavenly moments. It is a book to keep for reference!"

Rev. Dr. Lyn Hammond-Gray
Vice President, Universal Brotherhood University
Atlanta, Georgia

"Congratulations on such a wonderful book. I don't think there is anything like it, as it is so personal and inspiring about what living a Reiki-dedicated life can be like. How very inspiring and so full of the wisdom Shalandra has to offer."

Jan Dymond
Second Degree Reiki Practitioner
Corvallis, Oregon

"I loved *Living a Life of Reiki*. It is the first Reiki book I have read that is good for new comers and beginners to understand the "heart feel" of Reiki. It is straightforward while showing how Reiki can be worked with daily. This makes Reiki more real. It is also a wonderful book for those of us who have worked with Reiki for many years. The heartfelt love and appreciation Shalandra shares is contagious!!! And there are times when we need to re-remember things—like the life changes that Reiki healing creates."

Rev. Robin Morini, Reiki Master
Administrator, Universal Brotherhood Movement Inc.
Coral Springs, Florida

"I see *Living a Life of Reiki* as an important contribution to energy medicine information and literature."

Marika Breckenridge
Writer/Editor
Maui, Hawaii

Shalandra Abbey

Living a Life of

Reiki

From Complete Healthcare to Ultimate Freedom in Day-to-Day Life

Healthy Life Publishing

Designed by Dagan Ray
Printed and bound in
the United States of America

Library of Congress Control Number: 2009933230

ISBN-13: 978-0-9841744-0-9

First printing July 2009
First revision February 2010
First hardcover printing July 2010
Second revision July 2011
Third revision October 2012

Healthy Life Publishing
Maui, Hawaii

The mission of Healthy Life Publishing:
Make Life Better

DEDICATION

To Hawayo Takata because I believe this book
was more your idea than mine.

*

To Helen Haberly for sharing your story about
how Mrs. Takata assisted you to complete your book.

*

To Phyllis Lei Furumoto for your important
responsibility of holding the torch of Reiki at this time,
and for your ever-caring friendship, patience and guidance.

*

To Mikao Usui and Chujiro Hayashi for making the gift of
Reiki Natural Healing available to those who choose to
help make this a healthier, happier planet.

*

To family, friends, clients, students and fellow Reiki
Masters for your love, support, encouragement and Reiki.

*

To those who find Reiki and practitioners who use it more
because of reading this book. Thank you for making the
efforts in writing it worthwhile.

*

To the energy that Dr. Usui named Reiki. May your
treasures continue to be discovered and your precious
jewels forever appreciated and respected.

ACKNOWLEDGMENTS

Writing a book is a unique experience that involves a devoted community of diverse, caring individuals who believe in you and what you are doing. So many people help along the way, there are not enough pages to thank each one personally.

Gratitude goes to clients, students, colleagues, friends and family who suggested this book needed to happen in the first place. Thank you for your ongoing, untiring contribution to its publication. You all know who you are; without your continual inquiries, input, trust in me and Reiki, none of these words would have been written.

I also want to express my gratitude to students in the photos, all the people mentioned in the stories, and the many clients and students who so happily submitted the Reiki Success Stories in the last chapter. You contributed to my life and this work in a way no other person could. You will never know what a special gift you have provided for me in my life and for those who will see your photo and read your words.

Two key people who were most devoted and provided months of continual, non-tiring support and encouragement were students and chief Reiki writers, editors and fellow practitioners, Stefanie Hart-Neidenberg, Reiki Master, Denver, Colorado and Lisa Yocum, Second Degree practitioner, Kauai, Hawaii. Their many hours of faithfully supporting this new, challenging and exciting Reiki venture supplied much needed participation and encouragement to reach our goal of published completion. Thank you both so much.

Special gratitude to editor and Reiki angel Dagan Ray. I

couldn't have asked for better energy to assist in bringing forth my first Reiki book: *"Living a Life of Reiki."*

Gratitude is expressed to Celia Zagars for her radiant photography contribution. Who would have thought that photo shoots would be fun?

To Jim in Hot Springs Village, Arkansas who persistently, for many months, was ready to purchase the first copy. If for no other reason this book needed to be completed for you.

May Reiki energy bring back to all of us the energy we have sent out in unconditional love and caring through these pages.

TABLE OF CONTENTS

TABLE OF CONTENTS

Three – Reiki Treatments (cont.)

Four – Reiki Training   85

TABLE OF CONTENTS

TABLE OF CONTENTS

Life isn't about fear — it's about being willing to take on something new to learn.

INTRODUCTION

Two of the first questions people ask me about Reiki Natural Healing are, "What is Reiki?" and "How does it work?"

Reiki (pronounced Ray-Key) is frequently called Energy Medicine and is used by millions of individual practitioners as well as doctors and nurses in hospitals and other healthcare facilities across the country, including the United States Department of Veteran's Affairs. The following passage is posted at the Veteran's Affairs website:

> Reiki is another type of energy healing. The Reiki practitioner's hands are either lightly touching the patient's body or are held slightly over it. Energy is thought to flow through areas most in need of healing. In Reiki, the energy is thought to come from the Universe, and the practitioner helps to transfer this positive, healing energy to the recipient. The concept is bizarre to some, but people who receive Reiki often have positive experiences.

When Reiki practitioners speak of energy in this case, we are speaking of it in the way ancient civilizations defined it. We are referring to the life force that flows through our bodies, supporting optimal health, development, healing and fulfillment. This energy is what animates and enlivens all living beings. As Starr Tendo, a Maui newspaper writer explains: "Simply put, it is the energy that makes the world go round, the stars shine, the flowers grow, the child laugh and the waves of the South Shore break."

In a Reiki Natural Healing treatment session, the flow of Reiki energy simply encourages the body's own innate ability to heal and stay healthy. After a person is initiated into Usui Shiki Ryoho (Usui System of Reiki), the therapeutic energy flow is automatic and continual. The last chapter of this book is filled with testimonials of actual case histories where people have experienced Reiki healing with anything from broken arms to deep emotional and psychological issues.

Because Reiki is one of the fastest growing energy healing practices, more and more scientific studies are being conducted and research projects funded as Reiki continues to be integrated into our various health care systems. Some of the documentation of this work, which better answers the scientific questions of "what" and "how," is available at my website and can be read here: www.reikihawaii.com/reiki-research

A Brief History

Reiki Natural Healing was brought to the Western World in 1936 by Hawayo Takata, a Japanese woman born in a sugar cane camp on the island of Kauai who required surgery. As was custom of the time, she was sent to her ancestral home in Japan for the operation. But instead of receiving surgery she was healed by Reiki and returned to Hawaii with the gift of natural healing.

While living in Hawaii, Mrs. Takata was contracted to teach Reiki at the University of Hawaii on the island of Oahu and had Reiki Energy Medicine approved in the mid seventies by the American Medical Association to be practiced in Hawaii hospitals.

Hawayo Takata was the third Grand Master of the Usui System of Reiki. Before she made her transition in December of 1980, and after sharing Reiki for more than forty years, she passed the lineage to her granddaughter, Phyllis Lei Furumoto. More of this story is told in chapter two.

Sharing My Journey

At the age of fourteen, I remember watching my mother die in the hospital. Day after day as I went to visit I couldn't help myself from thinking, "There has got to be another way to heal." This experience planted a seed deep inside of me. A seed that wouldn't sprout and grow until much later in life.

My introduction to Reiki began in 1988 as a series of synchronistic events that would forever change my life. After many years of working for a living, I felt I had accomplished all of the goals that society promised would bring happiness. I was astonished to discover that something was missing. While searching for this "something," a co-worker at IBM suggested I make an appointment for a Reiki treatment. Not understanding anything about Reiki Natural Healing, I was surprised when something deep inside of me validated that the timing was right to experience Reiki. This something did not allow me to use the analytical mind that I had become accustomed to using in my corporate workplace. This felt new but incredibly okay to me.

After the one hour Reiki session, consisting of a gentle laying-on of hands, I was relaxed and peaceful and amazed at the healing abilities of the gifted practitioner. I remember thinking how lucky she was to have been born with such healing hands.

Several treatments later she explained that anyone of any age can learn to do Reiki after just twelve hours of training. In a state of suspected disbelief, I quickly registered for the next class. Since that first class encounter in 1988, my life continues to be healthier, happier and filled with exciting, and sometimes even, surprising events.

For over twenty years now, I have been living an extraordinary life of Reiki Natural Healing—one I never would have dreamed of while sitting in my office as an IBM executive in the 1980's.

While each of the three degrees of Reiki takes a student into deeper levels of internal healing, it also creates immeasurable external benefits. As each new day unfolds amazing things often happen that I wouldn't even think about, and all I can do is fasten my energetic seat belt and hold on.

In 1991, after I quit my corporate job and became a Reiki Master, there were only a handful of books on the subject. Today, you can find Reiki books everywhere, yet I still have not found anyone who has shared what it is truly like to live the life of Reiki. This to me is the real pearl in the oyster of our practice. Using Reiki on a continual basis throughout each day helps keep us connected to the source energy flow of life. This is where magic, in the form of improved health and happiness occurs, and along with it comes diverse forms of never-ending abundance.

What you are about to read regarding this ancient healing art, which I offer from the deepest part of my heart and soul, is a personal sharing of my long journey as a practicing master that is designed to move you progressively, chapter by chapter, to each step in the Reiki growth process.

It may be helpful to realize that this book is not a manual to learn this practice, but rather to give you a deep understanding of it and perhaps stimulate a desire for treatments and training. Reiki, as originally brought to the West, is an oral tradition and the ability to fully perform this ancient healing art can only be received from a Reiki Master in direct, physical contact with the student.

I have found that some of the more recent books on the subject seem to teach a derivative of the original practice handed down through a lineage of Grand Masters for more than 100 years. I respect these works for what they are, and also want to distinguish that there are differences in their modern approach compared to the information shared in this book.

Within these pages you will find a comprehensive study of the Usui System of Reiki and a path towards greater health, love and harmony in your life.

If you are already a Reiki practitioner, you will find helpful reminders and new ways to utilize more fully the precious
gift of healing in your hands.

This book will not only provide more awareness of possibilities available through Reiki, but can easily become a reference book for making positive lasting changes in all areas of
your life.

"In every culture and in every medical tradition
before ours, healing was accomplished by
moving energy."

Albert Szent-Gyorgyi, Nobel Laureate in Medicine

In this chapter we begin the progression of steps to mastering the Usui Shiki Ryoho (Usui System of Reiki). The journey of Reiki begins with an understanding of how energy affects you in your day-to-day life and what you can do about it.

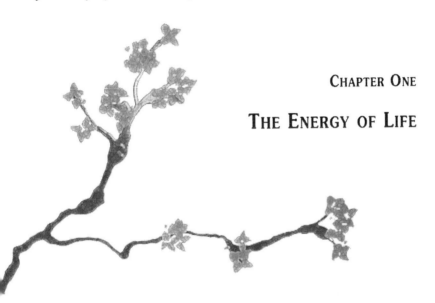

CHAPTER ONE

THE ENERGY OF LIFE

The source or cause of health comes from the energy that flows through and around an individual, rather than the functional condition of one's physical organs and tissues.
It is this energy that animates the physical organs and tissues as it flows through them and therefore is responsible for creating a healthy condition.
If the flow of energy is disrupted, the physical organs and tissues will be adversely affected.
Therefore, it is a disruption in the flow of energy that is the main cause of illness.

Once upon a time... our relationship with nature, through foods we ate, air we breathed, water we drank and animals in our lives, very naturally provided us with our basic connection to healing life force energy. Human beings walked and ran freely with bare feet upon the earth, allowing nature's life force energy to automatically flow up into and through our bodies. Food was consumed immediately after taking it from its source, while it was still full of this vital energy. We commonly gave gratitude to the plants and animals for they were considered our elders, teachers and friends. The importance of living in harmony with the flow of nature, the very energy of life, was not a mystery to us. It was a natural part of our every day lives. All of this supported our minds and bodies in healthy balance.

The Human Body

The human body was originally designed to maintain itself through the continual replenishment of healing energy in constant fluctuation circulating throughout the body. Time and again we see that the physical body has the ability to heal itself and stay healthy if given the opportunity. We are each blessed with a body that intuitively knows what it needs to function at its very best. The energies of our life environment interact with the energies of our bodies impacting positively or detrimentally everything we do.

Today, often without consciously trying, most of us have created extremely busy lifestyles that have disconnected us from what we need most to stay healthy and happy. At times we search the world to find health and happiness outside of ourselves, only to discover that it's not "out there somewhere" at all. The answers are simply, and have always been, tucked away inside of ourselves. Yes, we have heard this before but what does it really mean? What can we do about it? Why do we need to do anything about it?

The first steps to health and happiness are recognition and acceptance of what is depleting the healing life force energy in our bodies. We may be aware of one little thing or another, but when we take the time to bring all those things together, it can truly be an awakening experience. A new appreciation comes alive within us. It is one that may appear to have no easy solution until we can understand the simplicity of the divine plan.

Causes Of Ill Health

Although we behave as though inert matter were completely solid or dense, it is far more complex and spacious than meets the eye. When observed through a powerful microscope, we see that all matter is merely energy—a sophisticated cloud of protons, neutrons and electrons, the particles that together make up atoms. Atoms are organized naturally into elements. Each element has a unique composition of energy and a unique vibration. All matter is simply energy at a different rate of vibration than that of other matter and life forms. Understanding this, we can see that pure energy is the absolute basis for all forms of life and matter within our universe.

The human body needs to be kept filled with this energy of life to remain healthy. Energy is the basis for the apparent solid structures of the body and all that pertains to its anatomy as well. A seemingly solid structure such as a bone is actually a mass of living cells made up from atoms. All forms and activities of life, both anatomical and physiological, are supported by and simultaneously deplete the energy within the body.

When born we are fully connected to our source, "the energy from whence we came." This can be felt when the temperature of a baby's body is hot and their touch seems to soothe as nothing else can. As children mature, they are often gradually led away from this natural connection. It can even begin from day one. By not allowing an infant to be born in its own natural timeframe we take the child out of its natural biorhythms. The physical, emotional and spiritual bodies have an important need to develop fully in their own personal timing while inside a mother's womb.

Soon after a child emerges in modern day hospitals, newborns are exposed to vaccinations that many doctors still debate back and forth about the safety of. Newborns may also be deprived both nourishment and the precious bonding that ensues when a mother shares her breast milk with her hungry child. These factors can also impede the healthy development of the child's immune system, decreasing its natural ability to heal and consequently stay healthy. What this means is our natural healing abilities can be reduced before our parents even carry us out of the hospital.

Thus, the saga leading to the causes of ill health in our modern-day world continues. Many children today, sometimes starting at a very young age, consume manufactured foods containing little or no life force energy. Foods with high level of fats or sugar and lacking essential dietary fiber may lead to hypertension, high cholesterol and obesity. These risk factors, compounded with a sedentary lifestyle, can contribute to chronic diseases such as diabetes, cancer, asthma and obesity—not only during the formative years of childhood and adolescence, but also well into adulthood.

Reading store labels can start to create a course of healthy action in itself. Labels reveal to us that much of the canned and frozen foods are composed of chemicals and preservatives that are actually toxic to the human body. Highly processed ready-to-serve foods high in fats, sugars and chemicals are commonly eaten in today's world. Manufactured and processed foods don't contain adequate nutrients for us to maintain health. A guideline to make this process of reading labels easier is: If you can't pronounce the word on the label and don't know what it is, consider seriously not putting it in your body.

Animals today are fattened with steroids, given antibiotics and hormones, then are held in stockyards before being sent to the slaughterhouse. More times than not in our modern-day world animals don't run freely. We don't connect with the spirit of these living beings or extend an invitation for them to become part of our evolutionary nourishment, as was the practice of some earlier cultures. When we put food that has been treated with chemicals in our body it depletes our vitally needed life force energy, which results in creating more stress and dis-ease.

To further understand why there are so many sick people in our society today, consider the modernization of food production. Vegetables, fruits and grains are sprayed with pesticides, genetically modified, and picked before they are allowed to naturally ripen. Many of the nutrients, enzymes and natural flavor are lost during this process. By contrast, fresh fruits and vegetables grown organically in the backyard or purchased from organic farmers have vastly better flavor and nutrition. It can be an interesting experiment to do a taste test by picking fruit that hasn't been sprayed with poison or genetically modified. Then choose the same type of fruit that was chemically sprayed and picked before naturally ripening. Which tastes better to you? Which will nourish your body to support optimum health?

Our vital life force energy is further affected by modern advertising which causes us to believe treated and engineered foods are wholesome when they are not. Do you know about GMO? It is important information to consider as you pave the road to health and happiness. Genetically modified organisms are the by-product of splicing genes from one species into the DNA of another. A popular strain of GMO tomato combines DNA from tomatoes with DNA from a blowfish. Awareness of the dangers of GMO is imperative for our future health and wellbeing. These agricultural methods decrease biodiversity, add antibiotics into everyday foods, and introduce unnatural species combinations into our environment. More surprising information on this matter can be found in the book "Seeds of Deception" by Jeffrey M. Smith and the movie "The Future of Food" by Deborah Koons-Garcia and Food Inc., a Robert Kenner film.

What To Do About It

The cost of buying organic foods is minimal when compared to the ensuing discomfort of nutritional imbalances and medical expenses that can result from not choosing to eat organically. A proverb of Chinese medicine is, "Food is medicine and medicine should be food." Through making wise choices we preserve our health and well-being.

Our planet offers us a wide range of plant medicines through its herbs and foods. With the correct knowledge of how to use plant and food medicines, human beings have survived for centuries and have been able to heal some of our most serious diseases even in modern times. The body easily and totally assimilates herbs and herbal medicines. The therapeutic values are unsurpassed.

It is interesting to note in this context that the bible in Revelations 22:2 says, "The leaves of the tree were the healing of the nation." Herbs and herbal medicine purify the body, act as antibiotics against germs and increase both our energy level and life span. Many ailments we treat with harsh drugs can be addressed gently and naturally with herbal remedies, as well as with Reiki Natural Healing.

A great many medicines prescribed by doctors have serious side effects. We need to ask ourselves if these side effects are in any way worth the possible positive influence these drugs may have. Addressing lifestyle choices, diet changes and using medicines that are more closely related to plants and minerals from our Earth are all ways we can choose to reconnect with our source energy and keep us feeling good and naturally in balance.

Our Air And Water

On the same subject of maintaining natural balance, consider the fact that many ancient traditions recognize the breath as the most important sign of life. Have you thought about how we all share the same atmosphere and air? With each breath we connect ourselves with every other living thing on the earth. Pretty amazing don't you think? Deep breathing is an excellent way to enliven the senses and relax the nervous system.

Similarly, we are very closely connected to our sources of water. One thing that makes our planet so special among all of the planets in our solar system is the presence of water. Water allows the plants to grow, contributes to our weather and keeps our Earth cool enough for life to survive. We all share in this water supply for drinking, bathing, recreation, work and enjoyment.

Think about how air and water today are being adversely affected by human activity, further disconnecting us from the healing life force energy of nature and affecting our health on all levels—mental, emotional, physical and spiritual. Water and air resources, especially in metropolitan areas, are commonly polluted with wastewater, chemicals and factory outputs. Fresh air and water are essential to support and maintain health in the human body. Living in harmony with nature and the energy of life is not a luxury, it is a necessity for the health of our planet and future generations.

In many cities our water supply is fluoridated because we are told it helps to prevent tooth decay in children. There is now strong evidence that this is not true. In a 22-page response to the House Subcommittee on Energy and the Environment, Charles Fox (assistant administrator EPA) admitted that after more than five decades of fluoridation, at least tens of millions of Americans could be adversely affected by fluoridated drinking water.

Many people today are purchasing their drinking water. Who would have thought just a few years ago that we would be going to market and paying money for water in plastic bottles? The thought of having water delivered to our residence creates laughter among some old timers who once relied upon rainwater catchment systems to provide their daily water supply. In some parts of the world families continue to rely upon water catchment systems. Unless we are able to decrease air and water pollution these catchment systems may no longer be viable due to contaminated rainwater.

Within the last few decades drinking from both tap water and natural water sources such as lakes and streams is rapidly becoming unhealthy because of contamination. While the pollution of our planet is not an uplifting topic, the more we allow ourselves to become aware of these challenges born of unhealthy influences, the sooner we will desire to make changes supportive of our health and well-being.

Water is a precious and sensitive element. New study shows that water responds dramatically to our thoughts and intentions. Revolutionary water research conducted by internationally renowned Japanese scientist Masaru Emoto contains fascinating results illustrating how the energy of water and food can be affected. Dr. Emoto created a method of photographing water's crystalline structure as it is frozen. He then compared the crystals from water samples around the globe, finding extraordinary differences amongst various locations. His experiments further document water's response to thought forms. Some water samples were treated with loving thoughts, while others were treated with hateful thoughts. His photographs were astonishingly revealing. The love energy bottles reflected exquisite flower-like patterns, while the hate energy bottles showed a chaotic and disorganized configuration. Dr. Emoto has published books and photographs about his water energy research.

Dr. Emoto tells us that we began life as fetuses being 99 percent water. At birth we are 90 percent water. By the time we reach adulthood our water composition is about 70 percent. If we die of old age we will probably be about 50 percent water. What this shows is that throughout our lives we exist mostly as water.

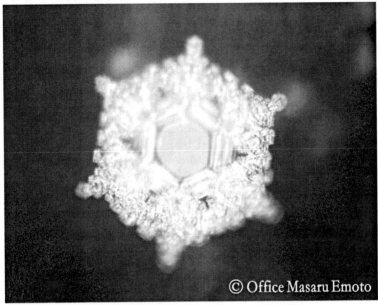

Water crystal treated with loving thoughts

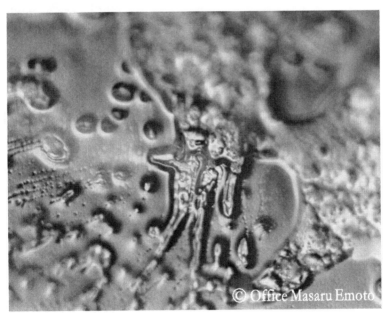

Water crystal treated with hateful thoughts

Since our bodies are made up of certain densities of flowing energy and about 70 percent water, it makes sense to consider just how deeply we are affected through continual exposure to environmental influences that disturb and deplete our priceless energy. This is important awareness. By continually living in the flow of Reiki Natural Healing we can improve the flow of energy in our lives and achieve optimum health.

Electronic Devices

Our natural ability to stay healthy continues to be in jeopardy simply by turning on television. When we search for entertainment, we often find programs filled with violence and bloodshed. Guns, reckless driving and the newest gadgets are pictured as being a way of life. Drug commercials, murder, plastic surgery makeovers and mischievous activities are pictured as the norm. These images on television and in movies easily affect our energy field and create various levels of ill health within the minds, emotions and bodies of children and adults.

To stay healthy today a person really needs to consider all the various contributors creating blocked energy and, consequently, ill health within our precious being. Think about all the new electronic devices being introduced daily. While flashy and exciting, how much does being exposed to them truly affect us? Keep in mind these devices can fill the time formerly spent enjoying nature while working and playing in the outdoors. It can be truly surprising to compare which activities in our daily lives support us to stay healthy and happy and which ones don't.

Recent research by the U.K.'s Health Protection Agency shows health concerns with some fluorescent lighting due to ultraviolet radiation. Overhead electrical power lines buzz above and around us. How could these intense electrical vibrations possibly be supportive to the flow of natural healing energy within our being?

Think about it: Rushed and busy lifestyles, foods containing chemicals that gradually poison the liver and weaken the immune system, unhealthy sweeteners, caffeine, drugs, alcohol, cigarettes, cell phones and computers all can be culprits creating tension, anxiety and illness around the world. Sometimes the technologies we think we enjoy and take for granted are causing us undue harm.

Sad but true, police officers continue to get cancer from simply doing their job using the police radar guns. Although much debate surrounds the impact of certain highly profitable technologies like police radar guns, the House of Representatives and Senate in Connecticut unanimously banned use of hand-held radar guns throughout the state based on pressure from police unions who insist they cause cancer.

When we consider all of the influences that our bodies have to process in the course of a day or in a lifetime we begin to ask ourselves what we might do to help stay connected to the healing life force energy that is so important for safeguarding our well-being. There are several adjustments we can make in our behaviors that support our connection to life-giving energy and that make us feel good about our health and contribute to a healthier planet.

Nature And Animals

Much about working with the natural energetic flow of life and staying healthy is learned by observing nature and animals. How relaxing it is to watch the flexibility of trees in the wind! Without flexibility they would break, but by being flexible and going with the flow of the air around them they are able to withstand the strongest forces of nature. Is there a message here for us?

Animals can help us to make this reconnection. They provide important messages by relaxing, exercising, stretching, eating only when hungry, drinking lots of water and living freely with the energy of life. Cats can teach us to relax and hang loose, stretch and exercise our bodies. Dogs show us how to be true friends and how to be aware of the energy of people coming into our sacred space. It is time for the human species to reconnect and stop fighting the natural flow of life.

Relaxation And Flexibility

While we are blessed with freewill there are times when it doesn't seem to be a good thing. How often do we give ourselves a day to do nothing and simply spend time enjoying the healing benefits of silence? The body needs exertion and rest in balance. Good health can only be found when there is an unobstructed flow of natural energy through a living system. Relaxing and being flexible helps to put us into alignment with the natural flows of life.

Continually we are faced with a complex world of information and experience. How we choose to interact with our world can be a blessing or a curse of freewill. Our senses are a gift given to us to honor and fill with beautiful experiences. The choices we make directly influence how our senses and health are lessened or strengthened.

Inner Knowing

We each have a priceless inner knowing that is constantly present to help us navigate our complex world. Over the years this inner knowing has received different names. Some relate to this inner knowing as coming from our inner voice or our heart conscience. Others call it a "gut feeling." For those open to its wisdom, this voice within is all-knowing and is without a doubt connected to our energy source. We can ask ourselves questions about the way in which we are living. How is this affecting me? As long as we don't give our thinking mind time to get in the way of the response, the inner self quickly tells us the truth about any situation.

Our inner consciousness is ever present and it is talking to us continuously, not just when we ask questions and not necessarily always in the form of words. For instance, sometimes the information may come in the form of body sensations like when the body sends signals in the form of a headache. This message may be saying, "take me outside, I need to breathe fresh air," or "give me some water to drink or nourishing food to eat." It is important to remember that there are basic needs that keep the life force-energy flowing in a healthy manner. When we do not listen to the body by taking a short-cut to relief, we may create more troubles and more critical body conversation. Our inner voice does not get quieter when it is ignored or numbed—it gets more urgent and persistent.

Reiki Natural Healing

Staying connected to the energy of life awakens a hidden treasure of natural abilities within us. By continually replenishing life force energy with Reiki, practitioners have the gift of ever-present healing energy that, among other things, automatically maintains a connection with the all-knowing inner voice. The practice of using this healing energy, called Usui Shiki Ryoho, is the system of Reiki that was entrusted to the Western World in 1936.

The word Reiki is derived from two Japanese words; "Rei," which means both universal in the sense of everywhere, and also spiritual wisdom; and "ki," which means life force energy, the vital force present within everything. Therefore Reiki can be translated as "spiritually guided life force energy." It creates and sustains everything in existence and can be used to transform, to recreate.

Reiki is also the one-word descriptive name for Usui Art of Natural Healing, which was discovered and developed more than one-hundred years ago in Japan through the dedication and experience of Dr. Mikao Usui. This art is an easy-to-learn, easy-to-practice way of using Reiki energy in daily life as a powerful transformational tool to promote expansion into a new level of awareness and being that restores health and harmony to the body, mind, emotions and spirit.

Because of Reiki's direct connection with universal energy, it brings us a basic consciousness that is able to provide exactly what is needed to restore life force on all levels. Reiki treatments work by dissolving and eliminating toxic energy and substances from various levels of one's being, whether it is physical, emotional, mental or spiritual. Then it encourages an energetic dance of healing energy within the body which brings forth a healthy environment to one's being. This makes it possible for true deep healing to take place.

With Reiki we are no longer covering up the body's messages, but addressing its needs to bring forth optimum health and happiness. Reiki practitioners and clients quickly learn that Reiki can be used and appreciated in any type of situation.

The Usui System of Reiki is a precise method of hands-on healing that uses the energy that is all around us and found in all things. As mentioned before, everything is made of different densities of energy. When we come in contact with these various frequencies of energies our personal energy field is affected and we respond accordingly on many levels. This creates an impact to our health. Intentionally creating pleasant energies in our inner and outer environment assists us to stay healthy.

You may know of people who understand energy, playing with it from time to time, having fun creating the perfect parking place or extraordinary weather for the day. These playful exercises that call on our abilities to work with the energy of life can be a fun enhancement to our wellness program as we learn to connect with and consciously use this energy to continually support ourselves throughout our daily and nighttime activities.

Reiki energy is sometimes called energy medicine. It heals

on every level: Physically by healing the body, emotionally by understanding and healing our feelings, mentally by curing negative thought patterns, and spiritually by helping us to love ourselves and others. Reiki Natural Healing encourages the body's own innate ability to heal and stay healthy. After a person is initiated into Usui Shiki Ryoho (Usui System of Reiki), the therapeutic energy flow is automatic and continual. The more we keep it simple and allow our minds to rest, the more the energy is able to flow to the top priority needed for lasting healing.

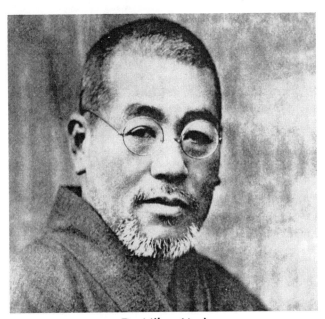

Dr. Mikao Usui

Dr. Mikao Usui developed Usui Shiki Ryoho back in the late 1800's in Kyoto, Japan, which is why today we call it the Usui System of Natural Healing. As was the tradition for sacred practices in Japan, when Dr. Usui came to the end of his life he recognized one of his students, Dr. Chujiro Hayashi, as the Lineage Bearer of Reiki.

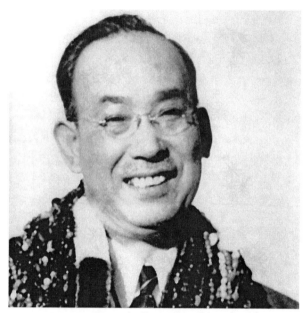

Dr. Chujiro Hayashi

Dr Hayashi, a retired commander in the Imperial Navy, opened a clinic near the Imperial Palace in Tokyo and kept records of his treatments and trainings demonstrating that Reiki finds the source of the physical problems and fills the vibration or energy need, thus restoring the body to wholeness.

In 1935, a young woman named Hawayo Takata came to Chujiro Hayashi for Reiki treatments and training. In 1941 before Dr. Hayashi's transition he recognized her as his successor in Reiki. In 1980 she handed the teaching lineage of Reiki to her granddaughter Phyllis Lei Furumoto.

We acknowledge and honor the grandmasters spiritually as our linage bearers, mentally as our teachers and emotionally as our companions in Reiki.

With Reiki, most anything is possible. Reiki's healing energy gives us the power to live lives of peace and integrity

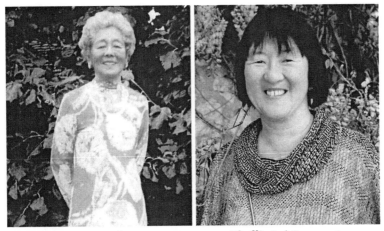

Hawayo Takata   **Phyllis Lei Furumoto**

assisting us to be healthy on all levels. The following chapters will show how...

"The next big frontier in medicine is energy medicine."

Mehmet Oz, M.D. (One of the most respected surgeons in the U.S. and the Director of the Cardiovascular Institute at the Columbia University College of Physicians & Surgeons, speaking on Oprah)

With a better understanding of energy in our lives, we are ready to gain a better understanding of Reiki itself. This chapter offers the background of the practice, its integration into the West and current developments.

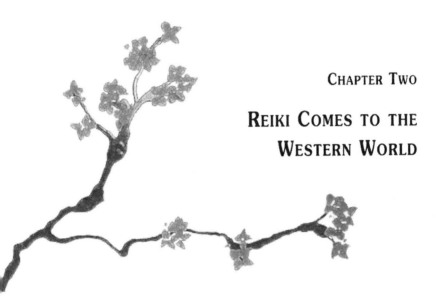

CHAPTER TWO

REIKI COMES TO THE WESTERN WORLD

Early one December morning in the year 1900, a tiny baby girl was born in the sugarcane camp at Hanamaulu, Kauai, Hawaii. She was so petite that her family and midwife agreed she needed to have a large first name to help her through challenging times in life. So it was decided to name her after the newly formed territory of Hawaii and the Big Island of Hawaii. She was given the name Hawayo (Hawaii) Takata.

As she grew, life was not easy for such a small girl who needed to work in the fields cutting cane and was expected to keep up with other children her age. Her frail body was easily overtaxed. One day she became so discouraged she got down on her knees in the middle of the cane field, raised her hands to the heavens and asked, "Please God give me something better to do with these hands than to cut cane." Little did she know the blessings her hands would one day bring.

In the 1930s her wish was granted. She became ill and as was the custom in those days, was sent to her ancestral home in Japan for surgery. It was not an easy journey. She took a small boat out of Kealia Harbor to Honolulu, then boarded a large ship and traveled for many days before finally arriving at her destination in Japan. Once there, the doctors told her she would need to build up her strength before surgery could be scheduled.

The Time Had Come

In Tokyo, she was on the operating table awaiting the imminent surgery. As the final surgical preparations were being made she intuitively felt that there may be another way for her to be healed. After inquiring of the head surgeon, she was told about the Usui System of Reiki and instead of surgery, she opted to visit the Reiki Clinic of Chujiro Hayashi. She remained there for several months while being restored to health and vibrancy.

After her remarkable healing was completed she asked to be taught how to practice Reiki so she could take it to her community in Kauai where it was so clearly needed. She was told by Dr. Hayashi, "No, this is not something that women do. Japan has shared its culture with the Western World before and they have abused it." Hayashi was adamant that this was not going to happen with something as precious and sacred as the Usui System of Reiki. Mrs. Takata, as it turns out, was as persistent as Dr. Hayashi was intuitive. He had recognized the war coming (World War II), and knew that Reiki needed to go to a woman for safe keeping. After all, Takata was Japanese and could take Reiki safely to Kauai. Following a lengthy time of proving herself worthy, Dr. Hayashi agreed to teach her Reiki. She lived in Hayashi's home with his family for one year working in the clinic and making house calls. Then after much practice she returned to Kauai to present the priceless gift of Reiki Natural Healing to the Western World.

First Reiki Practice

In October 1936, Mrs. Takata opened the first Reiki practice outside of Japan on the island of Kauai, Hawaii in the town of Kapaa. Next she moved to Hilo on the Big Island of Hawaii where she provided Reiki for some time before moving once again to the island of Oahu and practicing in Honolulu. Mrs. Takata spread Reiki's teachings to the mainland United States beginning with Chicago and then in the San Francisco Bay area. She later went on to teach classes in the southern part of British Columbia, Canada.

Hawayo Takata's persistence led to Reiki Energy Medicine being approved in the mid seventies by the American Medical Association to be practiced in Hawaii hospitals. She was under contract during this time with the University of Hawaii to teach Reiki on the island of Oahu. In her 44 years practicing Reiki she treated and taught many people how to work with the life force energy all around them. Today Mrs. Takata's Reiki seeds have expanded to almost every country in the world.

First Reiki Masters In The Western World

During the 1970's, after over forty years of practicing Reiki, Hawayo Takata initiated twenty-two masters to carry on the sacred Reiki teachings and standards she had spent her life upholding. Before her transition in 1980, two weeks before her 80th birthday, she recognized her granddaughter, Phyllis Lei Furumoto, as her successor.

These original twenty-two masters initiated by Hawayo Takata are:

George Araki

Dorothy Baba

Ursula Baylow

Rick Bockner

Barbara Brown

Fran Brown

Patricia Ewing

Phyllis Lei Furumoto

Beth Gray

John Gray

Iris Ishikura

Harry Kuboi

Ethel Lombardi

Barbara McCullough

Mary McFadyen

Paul Mitchell

Bethel Phaigh

Barbara Weber Ray

Shinobu Saito

Virginia Samdahl

Wanja Twan

Kay Yamashita

The Reiki Alliance

An alliance was formed among these masters, who decided to come together each year to share their stories and support each other as teachers of Usui Shiki Ryoho. The Reiki Alliance continues to meet annually and has grown to hundreds of members from many different countries around the globe. These meetings are a time of renewal, celebration and mutual support. For its members, The Reiki Alliance is a point of focus in Reiki. It is truly a living, breathing organization. Its form eludes definition as it is an expression of energy whose essence is movement. The Reiki Alliance website - www.reikialliance.com contains an international directory of masters available to teach and practice this sacred healing art.

Several Alliance members hold regularly scheduled Reiki circles. These circles are a time for Reiki practitioners to share the practice of Reiki with each other. As masters travel and teach Reiki throughout the world, the local Reiki circles provide a time of connection and renewal within the Reiki community.

Reiki Changes

Until about 1992 Reiki Masters in the Western World were teaching Reiki in a similar way. It was understood that the method handed down through the Grand Masters isn't for Reiki Masters to question—that it was not their responsibility. All Reiki Masters need to know is that they have a lineage bearer in charge of an oral sacred tradition and it is known from experience the system works. Boy does it work…

The life of Reiki Mastery certainly isn't always an easy path and yet the lessons learned along the way are always profound, complete and lasting. Time and again, as life begins to change, we may become afraid because we don't know what the lessons are. Sometimes we do know and feel tempted to run from them. Yet as each lesson after another passes, there is a feeling of being filled with so much humble gratitude and delight. There is an amazing fulfillment that comes from the education and the valuable understanding Reiki provides.

Beginning in 1992, as Dr. Hayashi had suspected, the Western World started to change Reiki and teach it in various ways. These changes created something new, a new vibration of energy. And yet they continued to call it Reiki. People started to question the system, asking for an outline of our practice. It became confusing for those looking for Reiki, as vital aspects were removed and new ideas added by different teachers. Today there are many different things being taught under this name that have little to do with the simple, sacred, dependable, healing art that was entrusted to us from Japan. However, my confidence in Reiki is enough to know that everyone receives what is right for him or her personally and that we merely need to listen to our inner-selves for guidance.

Office Of The Grand Master

As changes in Reiki began to appear, the lineage bearer of Reiki, Phyllis Furumoto together with Paul Mitchell, another of Takata's masters, formed The Office of the Grand Master and today continue to hold Reiki intensives for Reiki practitioners who wish to renew or become acquainted with the essential form of the Usui System of Reiki. For further information on these offerings, The Office of the Grandmaster's website is: www.usuireiki-ogm.com.

Personal Connections To Reiki Heritage

In 1990, while on the one hand I was very nervous about leaving the IBM Corporation and moving west to Hawaii to live the life of Reiki, I was also gifted with many validations regarding my decision. Having visited the islands before, my thought was that I wanted to live on Kauai, but I needed some kind of sign to be sure I was on the right track. Leaving behind the lifetime collection of my material possessions that were loaded in a 20-foot container in Miami, I took a plane to the Big Island of Hawaii, the southern most island. Not knowing anyone in the area, I requested the freight company hold my shipment until I knew where I was going to live. Like a young girl just out of school, I felt so much joy as I explored each island, visiting the tourist and non-tourist sites, meeting local people as we talked story about their islands, all the while making my way up the island chain. Kauai is the oldest of the seven Hawaiian Islands and located the furthest to the north, so it was my last stop. As the airplane wheels touched the ground I knew I had arrived at my new home. Kauai embraced me with open arms and didn't let go. It has been a profound love relationship.

Forgetting that Reiki had been first practiced in the Western World in the town of Kapaa, it was exciting to find myself settling there out of all the towns in Hawaii from which to choose. When the remembrance set in, it was at a much needed time, providing an incredible assurance that I was in the right place doing the right thing.

It had been ten years since Hawayo Takata had passed away and Reiki wasn't discussed openly very much on Kauai. I had to make a conscious effort to connect with its energy from the past. Finally remembering that Takata Sensei started practicing Reiki on the island during October 1936, I went to our local community college and read through the records of the old Garden Island newspapers. In those days there was only one small paper printed a week so it wasn't too difficult. This is where I located the first display ad for Reiki in the Western World (shown on the next page).

As my Reiki practice grew, clients, students and people I had never met, started to call and wanted to share stories of the lady who brought this form of natural healing to the west. It was fun to sit and "talk story" with some of the old timers about Hawayo Takata and her Reiki practice. I'll never forget one man who excitedly explained, "She was a real go-get-um lady, one of the first women to drive an automobile on Kauai." Another lady enjoyed telling me about her golf days with Mrs. Takata, sharing that she always wore white on the golf course, and that when she traveled to teach Reiki, students were asked to set-up tee times for her while she was there. I was told that as late as 1974, when she was 74 years old, she played nine holes of golf daily and when at home participated in 18-hole tournaments. One lady even called and invited me over to see her dining room set Mrs. Takata had gifted her with before moving to Hilo.

Looking back, I have to chuckle as I remember myself as the type "A" ex-IBM executive with white skin, blue eyes and

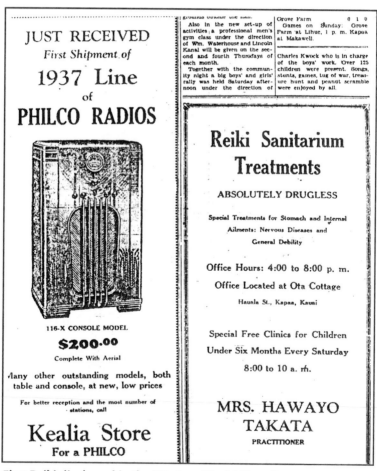

First Reiki display ad in the Western World Hawaii newspaper 1936

blond hair, attempting to "refine her energy" and learn humility. I was craving to know about Reiki's history in the islands, all the while introducing a method of natural healing to a tremendously multi-cultured, laid back, island society. Talk about initiations! Many more were coming in to me than what I was giving out. These kinds of life initiations are happening to this day and will never end...Reiki continues to be my teacher in the classroom of life.

"Health is a state of complete harmony of the body, mind and spirit. When one is free from physical disabilities and mental distractions, the gates of the soul open."

BKS Iyengar

Treatments give our body the energy it needs to heal itself. In this next step on the Reiki path to Freedom, we learn about hands-on, mini-, self- and distant treatments in a variety of applications.

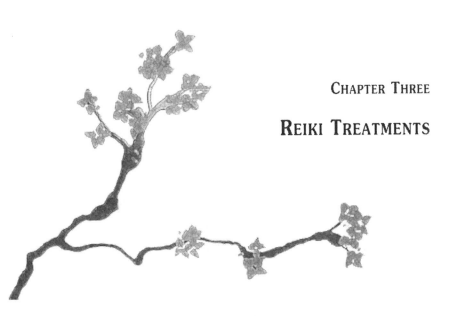

CHAPTER THREE

REIKI TREATMENTS

Reiki

Universal Life Force Energy,
An ancient gift from above;
Radiates from out the hands
Applied to each with love.
We are but the circuit
to help the body mend.
It's not us who stand as healers;
It's the energy we send.
Our Reiki hands stand ready
For what service they may do;
For when we're helping others,
We feel a healing, too.

By Greg Goodson, Reiki Master
Red Bluff, California

R eiki Natural Healing may be experienced two different ways, in the form of treatments or through training. Both First and Second Degree Training normally consists of individual twelve-hour classes for each with a Reiki Master. Later, some people continue deeper into the Reiki world with the minimum one-year training essential for Masters. For many people, treatments provide their first experience of Reiki and so it is there where we begin our journey into understanding the Usui System of Reiki.

Hands-On Reiki Treatments

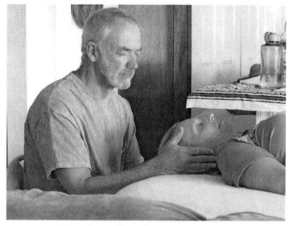

One hour hands-on treatment

Hands-on Reiki treatments are truly a divine gift! Treatments allow the body to relax in order to absorb as much life-force energy as possible. It is so comforting to have the gentle, soothing touch of Reiki hands assisting the body, mind and spirit into its highest state of wellness. In most cases, Reiki's healing energy is a delightfully relaxing experience. It allows you to unwind at levels you may have never thought possible, all the while enjoying the feeling of deep peacefulness.

There are, however, times when this is not the case. Reiki is also used to heal the cause of blocked energy located in the physical body, mind or spirit, not just the effect. This is different than just bringing temporary relief to a symptom. Sometimes going to this deeper place of healing can be somewhat uncomfortable.

While receiving one of my first Reiki treatments I cried throughout the entire session without any idea why I was crying. I'm not just talking about a few drops of tears. It was a continual, heavy, flow of bawling. I just couldn't hold it in any longer. Remembering my feelings as I was walking away from the treatment brings a warm smile to my face. All I could think about at the time was that I had been there for over an hour and paid money to lie on a table and cry. When I went home that evening I had an incredibly deep calming night's sleep and I awoke feeling better than I could ever remember feeling before. I felt like a huge weight I'd been carrying around had been lovingly lifted, leaving me feeling like a new person. I knew that something profoundly significant and real happened to me, but at the time I couldn't quite understand what it was.

Later, I realized I had experienced a connection to our divine source. In that moment, I understood more clearly another piece of the universal meaning of life and the cause of my emotional release during my treatment. I had connected with a level of love energy that I had not previously experienced. During childhood my family did not do a lot of touching or sharing of emotions. I had never realized how this had influenced me as an adult.

People of all ages from the very healthy to the very ill and everywhere in between can benefit from Reiki treatments. The healing energy goes to balance organs and glands, muscles and bones, etc., as well as the energy systems of the body. Reiki treatments simply fill the body with healing universal life force energy, amplifying our own innate ability to heal and stay healthy. We can never hurt anyone or give too much Reiki, because the recipient's body regulates the amount it receives, automatically sending it to the physical or emotional priority needed for their body's own individual healing process.

You hear a lot about "pain control" these days. Clients sometimes ask if Reiki can relieve pain. It can, but simply relieving pain is not always enough. Reiki wants to find the cause and heal the problem at its root, thereby eliminating the symptom of the pain. As Reiki energy works, hidden problems often arise which need healing before lasting results are achieved. When Reiki removes the cause, no effect remains.

If you think about the splendid completeness of Reiki's healing process, it can be hard to believe, but if you go inside there is an inner knowing present.

Often when practitioners start providing treatments there is a natural desire to make them "good ones." When we learn to get our thoughts out of the way and trust the healing energy, expectations can be released. We can know that Reiki is going where it needs to go as it addresses each healing priority. Hawayo Takata has been known to say, "When you are finished giving a Reiki treatment, you are finished because Reiki is doing the work. It goes by itself."

I couldn't help but laugh when a client who had experienced wonderful results after several treatments told me that Reiki works like an old U.S. Marine Corps slogan, "The difficult we do immediately—the impossible takes a little more time."

About 90 percent of my clients fall asleep before the first three of the twelve hand positions are completed. However, some need to release laughter or tears. Once in awhile, if a person has been taking a great deal of medication or drugs, the body may shake slightly as the energy brings the systems back into balance. It is important to create a safe space for clients to feel comfortable and free to allow releases to happen when needed.

Reiki practitioners and clients become quiet during a Reiki session to avoid interrupting the deep relaxation and potential release that may be taking place. Unlike massage, a good Reiki treatment is given with the client fully clothed, and you forget the practitioner's hands are even touching your body because the touch is so gentle and you are relaxing at such a deep level with the energy.

When Reiki practitioners provide treatments we understand that we are not the healer. It is the Reiki energy coming through that is doing the healing. We simply act as a vessel for this flow. Sometimes there is a sense that practitioner and client are one energy because in actuality they truly are. Takata Sensei told her students, "Don't try to tell God how to do His business."

It quickly becomes clear that no one can really heal another person. There are times when people need to keep their unhealthy situation for various, often subconscious, reasons. Reiki gives our body the energy needed for our personal level of healing, whatever it may be.

Very healthy people come for treatments as a maintenance program to help them relax and enjoy life more. Others come because they feel they have tried everything else, but are still on the highest dosage of medication possible and have yet to find pain relief. Time and again after Reiki they sleep calmly like a baby, which wasn't possible before the treatment.

Clients and students sometimes schedule ongoing Reiki treatments once or twice a week. Receiving treatments can help move our healing process forward more smoothly. As a Reiki practitioner it is a great gift to observe the steady healing progress enjoyed by these individuals.

One client came for Reiki treatments every Friday night for a couple of years. When I commented on how his physical and emotional body seemed very healthy and asked if he would like to cut back on his treatment schedule, he began recounting the details of his extremely stressful job and said that he hadn't found a better way to relax so completely after a demanding week at work. Before he discovered Reiki he would go to a bar and drink alcohol to unwind, which left him feeling terrible most of the weekend. Now, after his Reiki treatments, he wakes up on Saturday morning relaxed, full of energy and ready to enjoy his time away from the office.

I remember a clever story about a client who drank too much alcohol the night before an important meeting. Early that morning he called Hawayo Takata, our third Grand Master of Reiki, exclaiming that she must help him with Reiki to make it through his dilemma. She told him to come right over, then after the treatment charged him much more than he normally paid her. When he questioned it, she asked how much he had spent to get in that condition and then remarked, "Do you think this treatment is worth any less than that?"

Addictions

Reiki treatments can assist those with addictions, for when the body is kept full of healing energy it wants only what is helpful to function in balanced harmony. Smoking, drugs, alcohol, impure food, nervous non-supporting habits and more all naturally come into balance in the presence of the healing life force energy. In the case of an addictive problem, the practitioner will often recommend Reiki training. Then, when temptation arises, Reiki energy is immediately available for the individual to treat themselves and bring calmness and clarity to the situation.

Caregivers

Have you noticed there are times when a caregiver looks as if they need to receive healing more than the person they are tending to? It seems there are people in this world who more naturally like to give than receive, and of course vice versa. Well you can't get away with that with Reiki. The healing energy is continually working to bring harmony and stability to any unhealthy or unbalanced situation. As a person gives a Reiki treatment they receive the benefits of the energy coming through them before the person they are treating, and there is no transference of personal energy. Reiki is truly a divine gift to someone like a caregiver who may provide service to several different people during the day. Reiki not only allows them to help others, but to receive the healing benefits as well.

In 1992, during the aftermath of Hurricane Iniki, we provided Reiki treatments to the Kauai community. We had a continuous flow of people on the Reiki treatment tables from nine in the morning until nine at night. Even though we put in long hours, we felt great at the end of the day. I know this was because we simultaneously received Reiki during all those hours as we were giving it. Taking care of oneself is not selfish, it is practical. An empty vessel has nothing to offer. Reiki is a way to keep your container full and overflowing with little effort or time. It offers tremendous benefits to caregivers.

Childbirth

Painless childbirth without medication is possible, reports a Reiki Master couple from Germany. Their baby was conceived in Reiki energy and continued to receive it daily from the mother's self-Reiki, as well as hands-on treatments from the father and their students. Several others sent distant Reiki treatments throughout the pregnancy. At the time of delivery, the baby arrived peacefully into the world supported by Reiki hands.

There are numerous noteworthy Reiki stories related to childbirth. Using Reiki during the birthing process helps to decrease fear for mother, father, family and friends. Labor discomfort is eased with normally less medication needed, resulting in an overall smoother birthing and recovery process for all concerned. An ideal situation exists when a couple practices Reiki even before the child's conception. The baby starts life in the presence of the supportive healing energy. Receiving treatments throughout each stage of the growth process while in the womb, the baby's development is gently assisted and supported. Additionally, the expectant mothers who receive Reiki Natural Healing are healthier and more relaxed, able to enjoy their pregnancy and recovery time to the fullest.

It is an awesome experience to be in the delivery room with other Reiki practitioners all providing compassionate energy as a baby is born into the world. I love to hold my Reiki hand over the baby's spine and feel the healing energy naturally moving it into alignment. What an encouraging, comforting way to welcome a new being into our world!

The significance of this strikes a personal chord in me, as I had a caesarean birth and my spine did not receive the natural alignment that occurs in the birth canal. Consequently, it has been a lifetime challenge to keep my spine as aligned as possible in order to prevent pain from pinched nerves. With so many children being born through cesarean methods these days, I suspect people are going to have more structural misalignment and back problems. Many women opt for cesarean because it can make delivery more predictable. It is unfortunate that there isn't more emphasis on how important the natural birthing process is for the development of the baby.

I've often made the statement, "There isn't anything that a Reiki treatment can't help heal, if we surrender to the process and allow the time needed to do it." Well, a story in the October/November 2003 Reiki Magazine made me stop and think before saying this. There have been many reports over the years of women who could not get pregnant but were able to do so after receiving Reiki treatments. The story in Reiki Magazine told of a woman about thirty-eight years old. Having traveled almost ten hours by bus to visit a Reiki practitioner, she told the practitioner she had heard that some women have babies after they receive Reiki treatments. The practitioner replied, "Yes, this is true. I have treated three or four women who were told they could not have babies, and after Reiki treatments, they had babies." The woman agreed to a series of treatments. Three treatments later the practitioner said, "Maybe the problem is with your husband. Did you think about this?"

The lady responded, "Husband? I have no husband."

"Well then with your boyfriend?" The practitioner asked.

"No, no boyfriend," she said, "I live with my mother."

"Then how will you get a baby?" Asked the now bemused Reiki practitioner.

"I came to get Reiki treatments so I can get a baby." She said, "That's why I'm here."

The practitioner smiled. "Reiki is very powerful," she said, "it can do many things, but it cannot do this for you. If you want a baby, you have to have a man too!" The woman had lived with her mother in an isolated village and really had no idea about this. It's hard to believe, but it's true!

Children

Children usually adore Reiki treatments. They are naturally sensitive to energy and touch and know right away what feels good to them and what doesn't. I usually have a small toy available for younger children to settle them down as the treatment begins. Mothers of infants can place the baby on the Reiki table and give them a nursing bottle to drink from while I am starting the flow of healing energy. Normally, it isn't needed very long. As the energy starts moving the child quickly relaxes and takes pleasure in the Reiki energy before falling asleep.

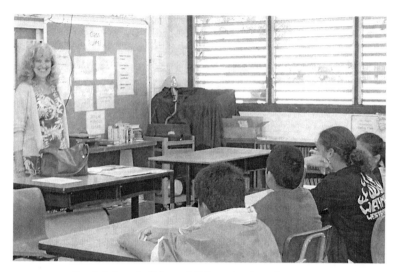

Explaining Reiki to children in the classroom

I love to go into our schools on the island and introduce Reiki Natural Healing. After an introduction while visiting our local 6th, 7th and 8th graders they sent thank you notes:

Kainoa said, "You guys are a good nurse...!"

Branden reported, "I really enjoyed Reiki, it was relaxing and soothing, I really want to learn Reiki so I can help my parents and use it on them."

Nahoku remarked, "It was fun...hope to see you again next time."

Ariel: "Thank you for doing Reiki on me two times in a row. Hopefully you'll see me and my friends come to your courses."

Dane: "Thank you for Reiki. It felt really good."

Brandee: "I thought that Reiki was cool when you guys did it, and I was shocked that it actually worked."

Chaslene: "I hadn't really known anything about Reiki;

just that it is healing of body. I learned a lot how energy helps your body. Thank you for coming."

Working hand-in-hand with teachers and parents of children who are taking Ritalin medication for hyperactivity can be rewarding for everyone involved. Recently I read that by the end of the year 2000 we were drugging more than eight million children in our public schools with Ritalin. Not denying that there are genuine cases of Attention Deficit Disorder (ADD) and Hyperactivity Disorder (HD), which are sometimes combined as ADHD, one can't help question whether these diagnoses could be correct for such a vast number of children. And if they are accurate, why are we promoting drugs that can create addictions while causing other health problems and not utilizing more natural healing methods? One of the highlights of my life as a Reiki Master has been my experiences treating and training children of all ages. It's amazing to witness the positive changes that start occurring in all aspects of their lives.

Animals

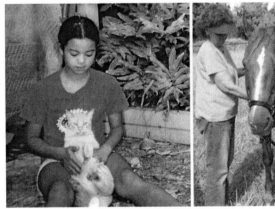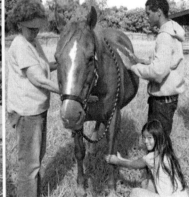

Giving Reiki to animals

Animals big or small are successfully treated with Reiki on an ongoing basis. My dog Malia always knew when someone had Reiki hands and she wouldn't leave them alone. Those without Reiki she didn't bother.

Here is a testimonial from one of my clients about how Reiki saved her dogs' lives:

"I am an animal lover so my pets are like children to me.

"One night I walked into our kitchen and saw a chewed up package of Mouse KILL, on the floor. With my heart pounding I picked it up. My dog Bella is a very mischievous fox terrier, especially with our new six-month-old puppy, Tilly, her sidekick around. We checked the dog's teeth and sure enough they had eaten almost two whole boxes. One dose (about quarter of a box), being deadly. We spent about four hours trying to help them. We had called poison control and the outlook for this type of poisoning was very bleak.

"At midnight we brought them both to the emergency vet. Tilly was almost unconscious. The vet was afraid they would not make it through the night. Early the next morning we called. They had to stay at the hospital, they had not improved much, and both were on IV's.

"We had heard about Reiki from friends of ours so we called Shalandra praying she could help our dogs. After the first session (a distant Reiki treatment) while they were still at the vets we saw significant improvement. Tilly began to eat on her own and their bodies expelled more of the poison.

"On the third day they were allowed to come home. They were still not out of the woods. Bella was completely non-responsive and would not eat or drink. It was danger-ous. That day it was time for the next sched-uled Reiki treatment.

"As I left the house, Bella would not get up or respond when I said her name. I came home shortly after she had gotten her treat-ment, and she jumped up and greeted me and even ate on her own. Tilly had an amaz-ing recovery even though it took a couple more Reiki treatments to get back her strength.

"We took them back for a check up. We had told the vet we had Reiki Natural Heal-ing done. She had never treated and had an animal live from this type of poison.

"We also had the animal poison control people call us back to document our dogs because they had not had animals live through this type of poisoning. A series of ten distant Reiki treatments saved our dogs lives.

"Shalandra never saw our dogs. They made a full recovery and every day my family and I are thankful to have them here with us today. Since this time four members of our family have taken Reiki training from Sha-landra and use it faithfully on others and ourselves."

Hawayo Takata worked for a long time with the cowboys at Parker Ranch on the Big Island of Hawaii. When the cows had calves, a much larger percentage lived after receiving Reiki. She also worked successfully with healing other farm animals.

Plants And Flowers

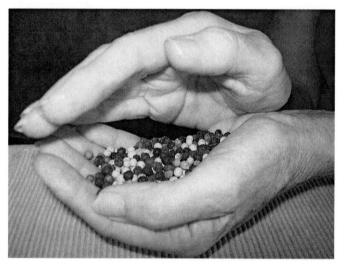

Energizing seeds with Reiki

When planting seeds, Reiki them before you place them in the soil and they will normally start to grow sooner, be stronger plants, and develop faster. Often practitioners pour water over their hand before it hits the soil and the plants adding more healing energy while assisting to purify the water.

Plants and flowers love the energy vibration of peaceful music so why would they not adore Reiki treatments? For longer lasting cut flowers we place them in water for awhile, then cut the stems under the water. Next we give Reiki to the stems, causing the water to go up towards the blossoms and allowing them to bloom longer.

In Hawaii you often see flowers in a person's hair. One of my students is a mail carrier. She kept sending Reiki to an orchid plant that normally doesn't bloom past April. No one

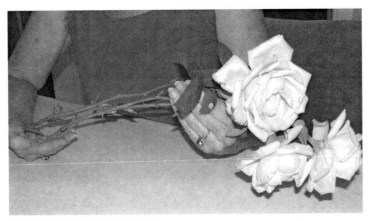

Giving Reiki to cut flowers will add life to the blossoms

could believe it when she continued into August to wear these orchids in her hair while delivering mail. Of course they were in more disbelief when she explained that she kept this orchid blooming with Reiki Natural Healing.

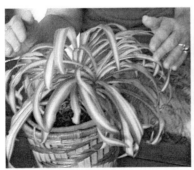
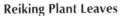
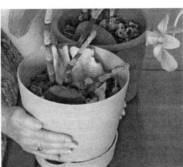

Reiking Plant Leaves   **Reiking Plant Roots**

Reiki can also be placed gently over the top of plants, or can be administered by holding the container to send supporting life force energy to the roots.

Stefanie Hart, at 27-years-old, was the youngest Reiki Master I had the privilege of training and initiating. During her year-and-a-half as a Reiki Master candidate she was a full-time student and received her Master's Degree at Naropa

University in Boulder, Colorado. Cleverly, there were times when she could work on her Reiki training and school projects together. An example was her master thesis in Environmental Leadership, "The Effect of Applying Reiki Healing Energy to Plant Life."

Stefanie's experiment involved three groups of ten green bean plants. One group received hands-on Reiki daily, another distant treatment, and the third regular care with no Reiki treatment. The seeds that had been treated with Reiki before planting showed increased germination rates and quicker development. Throughout the experiment the Reiki treatment groups were more vibrant, grew more leaves and were significantly taller.

The hands-on treatment group showed the highest rates for flower, pod production and germination. The Distant treatment group showed the highest rates of height and leaf growth. Vitality between the Reiki groups was very similar; however, it was improved over the Control group. If the data does in fact suggest a healing response in plants as seen through increased growth and development, than this healing effect may be reciprocal for both plant and human being.

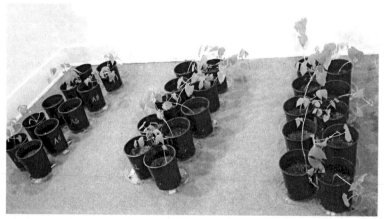

Research done on green bean plants shows significant improvement in growth with plants receiving Reiki (center and right).

The Phenomenological data suggests that applying Reiki Healing Energy to plant life creates a healing environment for the human experimenter through sensations of relaxation, sensations of a loving relationship with plants and nature, and positive self-regard.

The results of Stefanie's work were amazing and point to Reiki having a positive impact on the overall health and development of both plants and humans. Today, Stefanie is successfully teaching Reiki and providing treatments full-time in Denver, Colorado. The complete results of her experiment are posted on her website at www.ReikiDenver.com.

Food And Drink

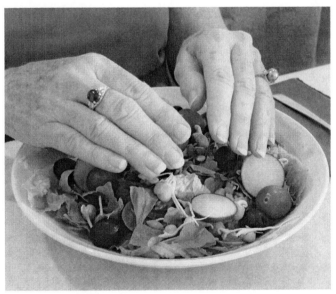

Giving Reiki to food before eating

Reiki practitioners find that adding Reiki energy to your daily intake of food and beverages helps remove energetic blocks caused by pollutants or harmful emotions. This not only makes the food taste better it also adapts it to the personal energy of your body. As mentioned in chapter one,

"The Energy of Life," much of the food we purchase today contains little if any of this energy so vitally needed for our health and well being.

Students seem to enjoy my story of being out with a gentleman for dinner one evening, when I just automatically placed my hand over my glass of water as we were talking. Soon he asked why I had my hand over my drink. I explained that I was giving Reiki energy to it. After I told him why, he asked if I would Reiki his scotch and soda, which I did while we continued our conversation.

Later, he took a sip of his drink and looked at me in disappointment and said, "Put it back!" He could no longer taste the alcohol! Further on into our meal, when this muscular man couldn't remove a tight lid from a small jar, I held it gently in my hands and sent it Reiki to release the blocked energy. Then I handed it back to him. He tried again to open it and was surprised when it popped open easily. Even though we seemed to enjoy each other's company, for some reason, he didn't invite me out again after that.

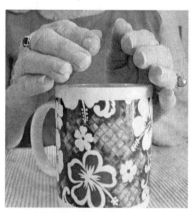 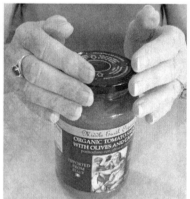

Giving Reiki to a drink   **Opening jar with Reiki**

One day in class, while recommending students Reiki their food and drink, I could tell one young lady was not able to comprehend any of what I was saying. Apples were sitting in a bowl on the table. I took one, cut it in half and positioned one portion on the table. I held the other in my Reiki hands for a few minutes while talking. Later I placed the two halves beside each other on the table. The lady was in total disbelief as she compared the colors, texture and taste of the two halves. The one half that had been Reiki'ed was white and crispy while the other had started to darken in color and was a softer texture. Reiking our food and drink also reminds us and provides the opportunity for us to have a moment of appreciation for what we are receiving.

Have you ever noticed when you walk into a restaurant there may be times when you feel happy and joyful, then following your meal your energy seems down? You may even discover a sudden feeling of conflict with whomever you are with. Believe it or not, you may have picked up the energy of an argument or something that was occurring in the kitchen and brought to you in the energy of the food you put in your mouth. Reiki life force energy given to food will assist to transmute the energy that isn't for the highest good of our body, mind and spirit. The results are experienced in a richer flavor, added nutrition, extra appreciation for the food, and a more peaceful and satisfying meal.

The benefits from eating healthy are endless! According to Dr. Nicholas Perricone, some foods can even help you look and age better. Our third Grand Master Hawayo Takata advocated a diet with many fresh vegetables and fruit. Her students reported that they would purchase huge bags of vegetables when she came to teach so she could make her favorite juice of fresh watercress, beets, carrots, and celery. She would tell her students that it was an excellent blood builder, which energizes the whole body and brings long, healthy life. It must have been beneficial, along with Reiki of course, because Mrs.

Takata had fresh, smooth skin with few lines and wrinkles on her face even at almost eighty years of age.

Medication, Vitamins and Supplements

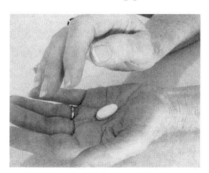

Giving Reiki to medication

Yes, Reiki, under a doctor's supervision, can help to reduce or eliminate your medication. But, what I'd like to talk about here is giving your medication a Reiki treatment. One student's husband had surgery and was told he needed to take a certain medication to stay alive. But each time he would swallow it vomiting would occur. This, as you can imagine, was a very unpleasant experience. One day out of desperation his wife held the pills in her Reiki hands before giving them to him. Sure enough, Reiki balanced out the energy and he could take the medication without upsetting his stomach. This will also work for vitamins and supplements, although they often are not needed after receiving Reiki initiations, doing daily self-treatment and eating organically.

Hospital Environment

Health care systems today are being challenged to provide a complete wellness package while at the same time remaining profitable. It is no longer enough to simply pay attention to specific diseases and trauma. Patients are now asking for health care that provides understanding of the total healing process. They wish to identify with the origin of the illness, the symptoms, as well as various options for curing and prevention techniques.

It is important to remember that hands-on healing as a natural form of medicine existed for thousands of years before modern science was created by the human mind.

Reiki is becoming the missing connection in today's overall health care programs, allowing more individuals to live healthy and balanced lifestyles.

In a medical environment Reiki can relieve anxiety and pain while strengthening a patient's immune system and overall sense of well-being. When patients feel better they experience new inner harmony and are more willing to participate in their medical healing procedures. Reiki Natural Healing is being recognized as an important tool to maximize a patient's care and minimize recovery time. Unlike complementary and other alternative healing techniques, Reiki is now considered an integrative treatment by the medical community because it will enhance any form of healing technique.

Hospice

Because of Reiki's healing, comforting, loving effect on both the caregiver and the client, it is being practiced successfully in hospice programs today. Most people are fearful of the unknown—they know the end of their life experience is coming to a close and yet they don't know what that means. This can be a frightening and lonely experience. It has been incredibly heartwarming to watch the changing facial expressions of someone in this transition after a Reiki treatment. Tenseness gently melts away and is replaced with deep peacefulness as Reiki energy connects the individual with the energy from whence they came while reducing the fear of returning.

Tom is a hospice volunteer on the island of Kauai and a Second Degree Reiki practitioner who shared this:

"I have only given Reiki to Kauai Hospice patients who have requested it. Without exception, those who have received it have benefited and been most appreciative. Also, without exception, it has been most helpful in assisting them with pain, appetite loss and sleep.

"Due to HIPPA regulations I cannot be too specific nor can I name the patients. However, one patient was in his very end stage of life or "actively dying" with body shaking, perspiring heavily and seemingly in pain. After about four minutes of hands on Reiki the perspiring stopped, his breathing became regular and his body stopped shaking. He indeed gained the energy that he needed to deal with his final hours in the body in a peaceful and calm manner.

"Another patient requested Reiki every time I saw him to help with his discomfort and pain from a facial tumor. After the treatment he was without pain and was able to sleep very well. There are many more instances."

Reiki Master Rebecca Henry of Lyme, New Hampshire shares:

"Reiki Natural Healing is a perfect fit to assist caregivers and patients. When someone is in the dying process it is all about letting go and the Reiki really supports that process. Time and time again I see how Reiki

facilitates and encourages the person to
relax, open and fall into a peaceful place
during the end of life process."

Debbie, an R.N. comments:
    "Whether one has days, hours or minutes
with a dying person Reiki is "soaked up," giving them ease of pain and fear."

For more detailed information and case histories on Reiki
in Hospitals and Hospice I highly recommend two books. One
is Libby Barnett and Maggie Chambers' book Reiki Energy
Medicine. An excerpt from the cover of Libby and Maggie's
book reads: "Reiki Energy Medicine is a fine introduction to
a technique which can truly enhance our capacity to make
our patients well. I wholeheartedly recommend it." – George
Remisovsky, M.D., OB/GYN.

The other book is Reiki: A Comprehensive Guide written
by Pamela Miles. An excerpt from her book reads, "Reiki is,
increasingly, being incorporated into modern medicine
because of one compelling reason: It works." – Larry Dossey,
M.D.

Health Insurance

As knowledge of the complete and lasting benefits of Usui
Shiki Ryoho (Usui System of Reiki) is spreading throughout
our society, insurance companies are integrating treatment
coverage into their plans. Health insurers are recognizing that
energy medicine treatment options can save them money. For
example, a series of several Reiki treatments costs much less
than surgical intervention. When surgery is necessary, Reiki
treatments before and afterwards have been shown to significantly reduce recovery time and hospital care fees. Under a

doctor's supervision Reiki treatments quite often reduce and sometimes eliminate the need for costly medications.

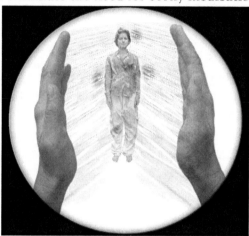

A mental picture of a distant treatment

Distant Treatments

Reiki treatments can even be given from a distance allowing the practitioner and recipient to be anywhere in the world. Distant Reiki techniques are taught in Second Degree Reiki training. Distant Reiki treatments are becoming more and more popular in today's busy society. What a gift to relax in the comfort of your own home and receive a healing treatment! You do not have to be in the presence of a practitioner to receive the benefits of a distant Reiki treatment. You can be anywhere, doing just about anything and still enjoy the pleasure and results of the treatment. Many people appreciate receiving a soothing Reiki treatment as they settle down for a night's sleep. These are sometimes the most effective because the more the body is relaxed, the more energy it is able to receive and utilize for its health and wellbeing.

Reiki practitioners often cherish receiving distant treatments in addition to their own self treatments because distant Reiki treatments work first with the energetic body before the physical body. Second Degree practitioners have the advantage of sending themselves a distant Reiki treatment. This is helpful when we are in places where it may be awkward or not possible to place our hands in the standard positions. Distant treatments for ourselves can often allow us to go deeper with our healing process. Practitioners support each other and their families in times of emergency like accidents or serious illness by several practitioners sending healing energy at the same time.

Distant Reiki treatments are also not restricted to one person receiving at a time. They are used beneficially for group meetings, animals, situations, events or anything we can dream of. These types of treatments have assisted folks to have more confidence while speaking, or while entertaining large groups of people, whether it is a special meeting or social occasion.

They can even be used to help clear unconstructive energy from our business or personal life, land, a home, office, car, or any type of thing or place. Supportive healing energy is priceless to send before, during and after surgery for both people and animals alike. Reiki can even be sent to situations to help heal issues from the past or clear away anxieties about the future. Because Reiki healing energy is "unconditional love from our source," it cannot be controlled and can only be used for positive results. The healing possibilities of Reiki are endless!

Mini-Treatments

After receiving Reiki initiations in First Degree training, healing energy flows freely from the hands. All we need to do is place our hand somewhere and there is an automatic flow of energy whether we are conscious of it or not. So why not take advantage of this gift by creating the habit of using it for mini self treatments continually throughout the day? As our body, mind and spirit are being depleted of energy we can eas-

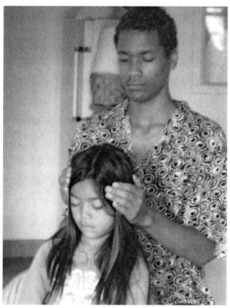

Example of a mini-treatment

ily and quickly refill it with Reiki's curative energy while we are doing other things.

When practitioners offer a treatment to someone that lasts less than an hour it is also referred to as a mini-treatment. It is usually administered with the recipient in a seated position instead of laying on a Reiki table, and normally last no more than twenty minutes. Mini-treatments are commonly used for emergency situations or demonstration purposes at Reiki introductions, health fairs or while volunteering at hospice, long term care, adult day care and at hospitals. Whenever there are several people requesting Reiki or when a person has a limited amount of time, mini-treatments are appropriate. Individuals will normally feel positive results from even a few minutes of treatment and may make comments that their headache is gone, or that they feel much more relaxed and calm.

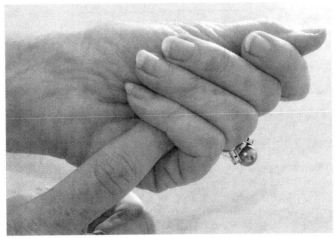

Giving self treatment for minor injuries

Minor Injuries: Cuts, Burns, Bruises and Bites

Mini-treatments are easily administered in times of emergency. Sometimes we jokingly call them "band-aid" treatments. Reiki energy amplifies our own innate ability to heal. The sooner the energy is applied, the faster we enjoy the results. For instance, when Reiki is quickly applied to a cut on the finger the healing process begins right away. Part of the energy's healing action may include stopping the bleeding and relieving pain, thus eliminating the need for band-aid coverage. I personally use Reiki on just about everything in my life and have not had band-aids, medication, vitamins or supplements in the house since 1989 shortly after my Reiki training. There are no guarantees with Reiki though and not everyone will find this to be the case for them.

The success I've seen healing bruise and burn situations with Reiki continues to surprise me because I know the painful results that normally occur. Immediately I place my

hand on the area, which in the case of a burn is not a pleasant sensation because it feels as if you are adding more heat.
The pain typically will intensify for a short time and then subside as the burn region begins to feel better and rapidly heal.
Time and again after applying Reiki there is little, if any, blister, scar or bruise from an incident—depending of course on
the severity of the injury.

One day while preparing to teach a Reiki class, I reached
over the tea kettle for a teacup thinking the boiling water was
turned off and received an intense burn on my arm between
the elbow and wrist. Students were scheduled to arrive shortly
and I needed to get ready for the training so I wasn't able to
Reiki my arm as long as needed. A nurse in the class said I had
received a second-degree burn. Whenever possible during the
days of training my Reiki hand was on the burn area. The
nurse was shocked to see, after only two days, there were only
tiny blisters in the center of a red area and in less than a week
the arm appeared normal. I truly believe if I could have spent
time needed to Reiki immediately after the burn occurred
there would have been no blistering and an even quicker
recovery process.

Insect bites and stings are dealt with much in the same
way. Students have heard me tell the story of a boat captain
who had a group of tourists out along Kauai's beautiful Na
Pali coastline. Suddenly, a passenger was stung by a bee. She
immediately started to panic because she was allergic to bee
stings and her medication was back at the harbor in the rental
car. The captain immediately explained about and applied
Reiki Natural Healing. The usual life threatening allergic
reaction never happened. The grateful guest claims that Reiki
saved her life.

Uncommon Uses For Reiki

Students are often in a state of disbelief when I explain

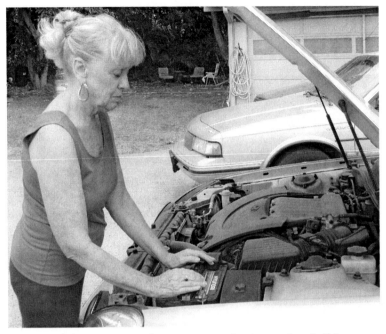

Giving an energy boost to a car battery using Reiki

that we can sometimes start a dead car battery with Reiki. Our Reiki Hands work as a battery charger sending the extra energy boost needed to remove blocked energy and start the positive flow again. A student returned to tell me the story of being stranded when her car wouldn't start. She said, "I remembered what you told us in class so I gave it a try and it worked! Now that I have my Second Degree Reiki and distant healing ability, if it happens again I won't have to open the hood to apply Reiki, I will simply send it from my car seat."

Reiki can perform in a similar fashion for other kinds of battery operated or electronic devices. It's fun to experiment using Reiki on anything that appears to be blocked and isn't flowing properly. Try it on your checkbook, wallet, clothes, shoes, jewelry, car, house, furniture and other items in your home. Before sending emails, greeting cards, letters, gifts and

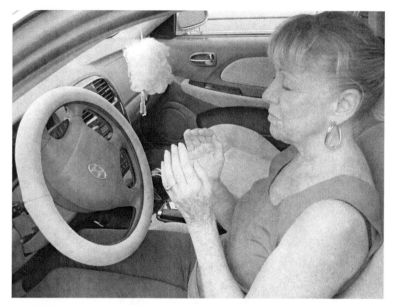

Giving an energy boost to a car battery using Distant Reiki.

paying your bills, give them extra loving energy with Reiki and enjoy the results.

Travel

Reiki self-treatment while traveling is an effective way to relieve stress, protect our immune system, and relax both the emotional and physical body. Over the years I have journeyed to many parts of the globe teaching Reiki. In the past, flight attendants and passengers would look at me strangely when I placed my hands over my eyes, ears, and back of my head. Some would ask if I was feeling okay. Today many flight attendants and passengers have been trained in Reiki. They usually just smile and later I may see them doing their self-treatment. Of course with Second Degree training we have the option of sending ourselves distant treatments while traveling. For long trips however the physical contact of our Reiki hands can be so soothing and comforting. Reiki gives us the gift of traveling for hours with often little to no jet lag. If the weather turns stormy or flights get turbulent you can assist to smooth out the energy of the air flow with Reiki.

Hotel rooms often come with various levels of blocked energy left behind from previous guests who have resided there. What a gift to be able to lighten the environment by assisting the clearing with our Reiki hands.

Healing Presence

Reiki can be used for anything and everything, bringing a healing presence to a person, place or thing. Experience has shown that the energy doesn't just come out of the hands but from the entire body.

I love this story about Gloria and Graham, a husband and wife from Western Australia who are Reiki Masters. They were visiting Hawaii and shared with me their story of a bus trip they took in Honolulu. In the habit of sitting next to each other, Gloria was a little surprised when her husband walked past her and sat next to a sad, unhealthy, looking man towards the rear of the bus. Later he explained his experience of feeling guided to do so. As he was sitting there he could feel the man's body pulling healing energy from his entire side that was closest to him.

After a period of time the sensation stopped, and he looked over at the man whose appearance had changed. He now looked healthier and more relaxed. And of course Graham was also energized by the unlimited supply of healing energy pouring through him. In Reiki classes, I love to share that all we need to do Reiki is our hands, but that no longer applies as this story demonstrates. There is even a Reiki practitioner who was in a car accident and lost both arms. So he then had his feet initiated and started giving treatments on the floor with his feet.

Reiki treatments are a wonderful way to manage our

health and help to bring all aspects of our life into balance. In the beginning of this chapter I shared with you about one of my first Reiki treatments. In the days that followed I was sure beyond a shadow of doubt that it was a positive experience. I returned over a period of about six months for more treatments. Each one was a different healing experience. All this time I had no idea that this was something a person could learn to do. I had assumed that this lady was simply born with an incredible healing ability. You can imagine my surprise when one day she suggested I register for a First Degree class. Following my excitement of learning about treatments was this new found joy of finding I could actually learn to do them. I quickly registered for a First Degree Reiki class.

"Reiki will bring you Health, Happiness, Prosperity and Longevity."

Hawayo Takata

Training provides a tool leading to health and happiness. This chapter covers the levels of training in the oral tradition, choosing a teacher and the many benefits of training.

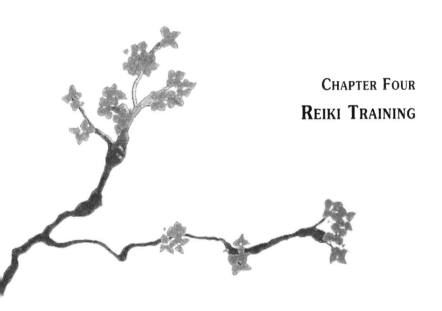

Complete Health Maintenance Program

Many people today not only desire, but are searching for a complete health maintenance program like Reiki—one that provides a means to feel better on an ongoing basis. People who have attended my training classes have been called to do so for many different reasons. Some have benefited from receiving treatments and want to pass along what they have had the good fortune to experience. A person may be ill or have a loved one in poor health and are searching for ways to help. Or there are those who wish to ease the pressure of being a caregiver. It's a simple equation: When we take care of ourselves we have more to give to other people.

Healthcare Professionals

Those involved with both hospice and hospital environments find healing for themselves as well as a renewed sense of purpose through the continual support they receive by learning and practicing Reiki self-treatment. Reiki helps them keep a positive attitude while easily and naturally sharing that uplifting feeling with those around them.

Individuals who practice other types of healing modalities are often drawn to Reiki for the protection this natural energy flow provides. Caregivers, medical professionals, massage therapists, counselors, etc., who are in constant contact with patients or clients may find they are experiencing to some degree the problem of the person who just left their office. There can be a transference of personal energy. When our energy field is full of Reiki healing energy, it is difficult if not impossible, for negative or unhealthy energies to intrude on a practitioner or their client. Reiki provides invaluable protection for those who practice it and for those who come in contact with a Reiki trained individual.

Any healing professional will automatically take themselves and their business to a new level of healing after Reiki training and practice. Reiki provides an easy way to do this because its healing properties enhance any type of therapy. One of the amazing things about Reiki is that it brings what energetic support is needed to any given situation. If integration of other therapies are needed or not needed, the energy of Reiki generally will bring that clarity. The more one practices Reiki the greater the personal and professional benefits.

Students Of All Ages

Students of all ages are called to practice Reiki because it is a natural way to stimulate energy and mental clarity. Although adults can certainly use this too, today's high schools and primary schools are a superb place to teach children and young adults healthy ways to manage the stress in their lives. Peer pressures from friendships, family relationships, sex, drugs and media, all pale in significance after learning and practicing Reiki. Students may simply want to be healthier and more relaxed allowing them to excel in school and every other facet of their life.

A Teenager's Reiki Story & Message

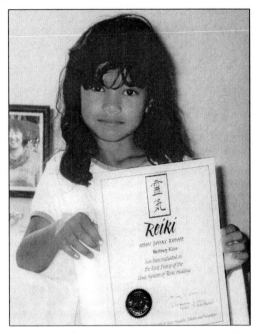

Britney Ellis, First Degree at 7 years old

"After Reiki Natural Healing helped me in my life I talked to my 7 year old granddaughter about it. She was interested in taking the training. At that time she was having a hard time with her grades and getting along in school. She couldn't stay focused in class and would daydream and not pay attention. Lots of times she would not complete her homework or other work assignments. The counselor recommended special classes and maybe putting her under the program for children with attention deficiencies. I just knew she could work through this and didn't need the Ritalin medication. She did not have a learning problem as tests showed. In fact she did superior in the tests. Maybe Reiki could help her.

Shalandra had a long talk with my grand-daughter and recommend she earn at least half of her class fee, which was $150; quite a test for a seven year old. We worked it out where each day if she was good in school she would receive a green card from the teacher. Each week I would pay her for getting green cards. For two months she received green cards almost daily and earned the money for her class.

It was exciting when she finally took her training in May 2000. Reiki helped Britney to settle down in school and not be so rest-less in class. It helped her improve her grades and not get sick so often. She had been getting sick a lot with bad coughs and congestion. In fact she became my teacher advising me about my driving, teaching me not to drink alcohol and coffee or smoke cig-arettes. She became totally against swearing. In this day and age many people find this amazing.

Tuesday night practitioners on Kauai get together to share Reiki with each other. Brit-ney attended these for four years even though she may have been tired or even sick at times. It was always cute to see such a small person giving or receiving the energy

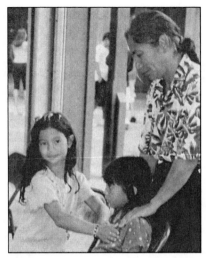

Britney practicing Reiki at a health fair

like everyone else. She also loved to go with the other practitioners to Reiki Introductions, Health Fairs and even help where she could at our Reiki Hospital program.

Reiki has helped her to participate in many different sports and given me the energy to keep up with my granddaughter getting her to all these activities. She makes friends easily and other kids look to her as a friend and player. At one point in time she was playing Soccer, Volleyball and Hula. If she had a bruise, sore arms, hands or legs, it was always the Reiki helping to heal her body. Reiki is a natural part of her life and in everything she does. She continues with her hula classes and her connection to nature and animals is great to see.

After a couple of active Reiki years it was just a natural phase for her discussions to begin about taking the second degree class.

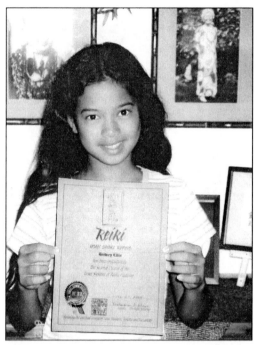

Britney Ellis, Second Degree at 11 years old

Again, she would have to earn the money and start preparing herself for the training. Shalandra worked with her on what was needed before she could be accepted for training; earning at least one half of the class fee, self treatments each day without fail, working more with the Reiki Precepts, and to give and receive more one hour treatments.

I was surprised when Brit told her Reiki Master that this time she wanted to earn the full class fee not just half of it. This took a little more effort to do her self treatments morning and night. This time I and other practitioners helped by paying her for one hour treatments and household chores.

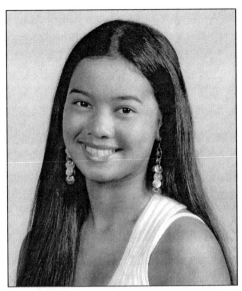

Britney Ellis at 14 years old

These ranged from washing dishes, washing my truck, folding clothes, putting out the rubbish and cleaning the house. I would also give her one hour treatments. So she really worked hard to earn the $500 dollars for her class. It was amazing to see the enthusiasm that she had to earn this money for her class. Boy, did she learn the value of the dollar. At 11 years old she was ready and completed her second degree training.

Each day I see more ways how Reiki helps Britney. She has an asthma condition that no longer requires taking medication every day. She hardly ever gets sick now with Bronchial coughs or Pneumonia eliminating going to the emergency rooms at night. She is active in sports such as Soccer, Volleyball, Hula and Track. She loves to swim and would like to be a cheerleader. Last year the first quarter she was on the Honor Roll list and the other three quarters she was honorable mention; a very big change from low grades.

She has more confidence and self esteem. Many have commended on her beauty and how well she speaks around adults. She asks a lot of questions and has a quest to know. She continues her hula and great love of animals. The only thing that stops her from all these activities is her grandmother's ability to keep up with her.

She is a lot more focused and now a role model for other kids. At the A+ program she reads books to the younger kids and has great empathy for kids with physical problems. When I get hurt she is there with the Reiki. At eleven years old she has so much to look forward to and do. The question to Britney was "what would you like to do when you are older?" I asked if one day she might like to be a Reiki Master. Look into her eyes and there lies the answer."

Britney's Essay On How Reiki Can Help Teens

Reiki has helped me in so many ways. I believe that it can help the teens. It can help them by controlling what is going on now days. For example: Drugs, grades, attitude, responsibility, health problems and sports.

Reiki can help the kids who are into drugs because it'll show their body's that they don't need that stuff and there are better things in life. It'll make their body not want these kinds of thing. Kids want to try it because

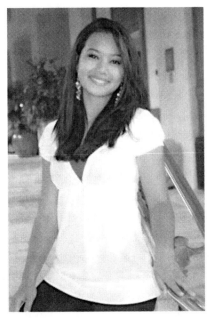

Britney Ellis at 16 years old

they think its cool, but it's not and Reiki can help with that situation. Reiki will give you a better feeling than drugs.

If kids are into drugs, I believe it'll make it harder for them in school how is it possible for them to concentrate on school? It'll make them not care about school and they might not even get to finish school because they're so hooked on drugs and school might not be as important as it use to be. I know for a fact Reiki can help kids in school, it'll help them be more focused into school work and not other unimportant things that can wait.

If kids now days want to play sports how can they do that with low grades? Sports are such a big deal for kids now days. Reiki can help them focus, help build their body strength, and it'll help with their school work that's needed to play sports in the first place. It would give them the perseverance to want to keep going for the sport even if they didn't want to.

Some kids also have really bad attitudes. I'm pretty sure if they were to take Reiki, their attitude would be so much better. Kids have bad attitudes because that's how they were raised to act. Or some kids yell because in their house they have to speak above others. If they were to do Reiki, they would be able to be calmer and not as aggressive.

Reiki can also help with responsibility; doing Reiki helps you put your priorities straight. Reiki helps you know what is right from wrong and can lead you to a better path in life. Help you be independent and want to accomplish something. It'll give you the energy to do whatever you want to do.

Reiki also helps a lot of people with health. It doesn't only help yourself; it helps anyone you'd like to share it with. I have asthma and I played sports and I really needed help and it helped me with my breathing and being able to cope with my asthma. I've seen so many miracles with Reiki, it's helped so many people with their health problems and they've gotten better within a short period of time. It was miraculous.

Taking Reiki was the right thing to do. Now that I've taken Reiki, everything goes into place now. And by following the Reiki Precepts, I get through my day with no problems. Reiki will bring nothing but good in your life.

Musicians, Artists And Writers

Reiki is also a creative energy. It can inspire students in both their confidence and creativity. For these reasons, scores of musicians, artists and writers are drawn to Reiki training. With Reiki's encouragement inspiration truly seems to flow. I have had musicians come to Reiki training and afterwards decide it is time to go public, cut their first CD, or play a new type of music. Artists are often motivated to investigate new mediums of artistic expression. Writers' words may move into entirely new directions.

Conception

Women wanting to have children can greatly benefit from Reiki's healing energy. As each stage of development unfolds, from before conception to raising a happy healthy child, Reiki supports and assists in the process. After learning self-treatment in First Degree training, the mother-to-be can begin preparing her body and emotions for the pregnancy, delivery and child rearing. Dad and the rest of the family can learn Reiki too, providing energetic assistance before, during and after the birthing process. For families and friends it can be a wholesome way to securely unite their bond by sharing Reiki treatments with each other.

Medicine

Our medical system seems to have invented a pill for just about everything. But while prescriptions may treat the symptoms of illnesses, they often don't go to the root cause of them. Because Reiki works on all levels—emotional, physical, mental and spiritual—and addresses the cause of the ailment, it can offer more lasting results. Reiki is medicine for the whole body because it brings you into alignment with the energy of the universe. For this reason, those looking for an overall health maintenance program, including both physical and emotional health care, find themselves enjoying the practice of providing Reiki for both themselves and their loved ones. Today a growing number of doctors and other health-care professionals are recommending a form of energy medicine like Reiki. Some Reiki hospital programs may be viewed on my website www.reikihawaii.com/reiki_links.html

Reiki Classes

Reiki classes differ from other classes you may have experienced. Students learn to do their self-treatments after receiving Reiki initiation, which is a ceremonial act that awakens and provides an automatic flow of healing energy. During a self-treatment, the student places his or her hands comfortably on his or her body to enable the flow of life-force

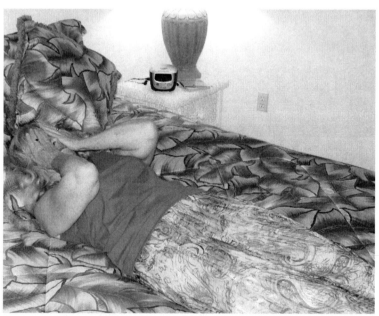

New students first learn to do self-treatments after initiation

energy upon contact. Specific hand positions are taught to get the most out of the process. Each hand position works off the energy from the previous one.

When self-treatment becomes a daily habit Reiki actually becomes a healing partnership. This trouble-free practice can actually change a person's life. Why? Because when the body is continually receiving healing life force energy, unsupportive habits that may have been fun in the past just seem to lose their appeal as they are replaced by those that contribute to our overall health and well-being. This natural course of action then causes healthier habits to become more pleasurable than old unhealthy ones.

Food And Beverage

Foods and beverages that are generally unhealthy, yet might be easy to indulge in, time and again seem to just naturally lose their taste appeal after Reiki training and practice. Reiki practitioners and masters who enjoy even an occasional glass of organic beer or wine often find the taste is dreadful if they attempt to consume it anytime they are close to providing Reiki treatments and training. Afterwards the desire for it normally has disappeared. One of Takata's masters commented that her master explained to her students, "Reiki and alcohol do not mix." They are different energies and Reiki is to be kept pure and not mixed with any other energy.

After Reiki some people may also find they are suddenly attracted to eating more organic raw foods full of life force energy and cooking less, as the cooking process diminishes much of the life force and nutrients from the food. Often we are guided to discover the fulfilling flavors and benefits of juicing fresh fruits and vegetables which can bring great improvement to ones energy and sense of well-being. There are also people who had sugar addictions who no longer crave the refined sugars in sweets, but instead find a new love of natural sugar in organic fresh fruits and natural sweeteners.

Addictions

More and more folks today are drawn to Reiki to help cure addictions of all kinds. As the old habits that no longer serve us dissolve away, exciting pathways open up for new possibilities. When the body is supported by and can easily draw from this healing energy it continues to restore itself to health and vibrancy on all levels—body, mind and spirit.

Drugless Treatment

Mrs. Takata, the third Grand Master of Usui Shiki Ryoho, has been known to say "Reiki is a drugless treatment for all conditions." Our second Grand Master, Dr. Chujiro Hayashi, has been quoted as saying "Reiki, upon contact, begins to revitalize and restore the balance of your entire system." After working with Reiki Natural Healing since 1988 I am in continual amazement at the power in its pure simplicity and how much wisdom each of the Grand Masters holds in their integrity with the practice. We may be moving into a modern era, but my experience continues to verify how vitally important it is for us to honor the system as it was handed down to us by our Reiki lineage bearers.

Levels Of Training In The Oral Tradition

Reiki is intended to be an oral tradition handed down by word of mouth to each student by the Reiki Master. Reiki Masters have received a minimum of one year's intensive personal training from her or his master and are continually practicing living the life of Reiki.

Traditionally, there are three levels of Reiki training: First Degree, Second Degree, and Reiki Master. Each is designed to be experienced during training, fully integrated energetically, and enjoyed completely before moving to the next. Those who have been initiated into Usui Shiki Ryoho and have surrendered to the simplicity of the healing process, by doing daily self-treatment and treatment with other people, will agree that the training starts with the registration for First Degree class and never ends.

When someone becomes a Reiki Master it doesn't mean the learning stops. What it does mean is that new lessons become part of an unending process continuing at just the right pace as the Master receives deeper challenges and benefits while teaching and learning to live the life of Reiki. Masters become an artist of Reiki as they create their personal Reiki Master picture without changing the form of the system.

The Right Teacher

When the student is ready Reiki will find them. Ask any student of Reiki how they found their Master and learned this healing art. They will likely light up as they tell you the story of the beloved friend or miraculous events that happened to get them to their First Degree class. The stories of how people find out about Reiki and the journey that takes them on their way to the trainings are endless. Those accounts themselves could easily fill the pages of an interesting Reiki book. When someone registers for a class they typically, though not always, have a clear intention and are ready to make positive changes in all areas of their life.

I will never forget the helicopter pilot who recognized he needed help with his healing process. One day as he was surfing the internet for a replacement part for his chopper my website suddenly popped up in front of him. After exclaiming, "what's this?" he read further, made appointments for treatments and eventually became a Second Degree Reiki practitioner. Not only did his physical and emotional health improve, he was surprised to find after flying helicopters for nearly thirty years, how easily the controls glided into gear after his Reiki training. Reiki energy will assist us and all things we come in contact with to flow more smoothly.

Students are drawn to the energy of a Master who carries energy similar to their own. When the connection is made there is often a feeling of excitement and anticipation. There is an inner-knowing that you could be comfortable with this person for a long time to come. As the student and master energy continues to grow together there is an innate understanding that it can easily become a lifelong friendship.

Class Registration

Reports have demonstrated that the moment someone registers for Reiki training, the healing energy begins preparing the student to receive initiations. Unhealthy things we have accumulated in life just seem to begin falling away, making room for the new. This could include emotions, habits, relationships, jobs and the list goes on and on.

There are stories of individuals who call and say they want to register for training but don't have the class fee. I suggest they find an attractive envelope and write First Degree Reiki Training on it. Then place it in a special space in their home, holding it daily between their hands and filling it full of their positive energy, while also seeding it from time to time. More often than not it fills effortlessly and when counted is just the amount needed for their training.

Manifesting the class fee may not happen in the timeframe one desires or expects, but it is always the ideal timing for that person's forward progression in life. Coming to the training this way, offers the individual a great lesson in grounding an intention, while moving through what seemed to be a limitation. They learn the invaluable experience of how to work with and not against the energy of life.

Reiki teaches us to allow an equal exchange of energy to flow in and out, out and in, not only while practicing Reiki

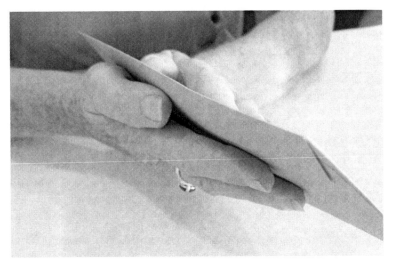

Giving positive energy to a money envelope

but in all other facets of our lives. As Reiki Masters we do not promote poverty consciousness by giving Reiki away. Its indescribable value and our self worth need to be understood and respected on all levels. Money is an important aspect of modern day life and our healing. That is why I have devoted an entire chapter to the energy of money—so more on this in Chapter 6: "Money is Energy."

Reiki Pathway

When one steps onto the Reiki pathway the enchantment begins. A charming man reported following his First Degree training that he felt as if someone had untied his hands that had been held behind his back all his life. He went on to say that after First Degree training he had the feeling he had been plugged into a continual flow of about 110 volts of healing energy. After going though a purification process, and many Reiki treatments later, his pipes were cleaner so more energy could come through.

Following Second Degree training he said he felt he was carrying 220 volts of power to work with, and that he couldn't wait to see what life would be like after master training. Because then, as he shared Reiki initiations, he would be receiving that energy as it flowed through him to his students.

Why was he experiencing this constant increase in healing power? It was because he faithfully had committed to the habit of self-treatment and the experience of giving and receiving full hour treatments with other people. He continually kept his body full of healing life force energy allowing his own healing on all levels while assisting other people in theirs. He now could see clearly that his choices in life were unlimited. He was free to be healthy and make decisions to enjoy life, following his heart's desire. Isn't that really what living is supposed to be all about?

My experience continues to affirm that the level of healing energy one receives from Reiki training is in direct alignment with how close we are to honoring the system entrusted to us in our classes. In Usui Shiki Ryoho training we teach that Reiki is an oral tradition and to keep the classes clean of non-essential material. If it isn't about Reiki, it doesn't belong in a Reiki classroom. When we start to change the system with something that seems insignificant, it means that on some personal level, we don't trust the degree of healing that is possible with Reiki.

This always comes back around to needing to do more Reiki on ourselves. Avoidance and denial are usually easier, so if we aren't careful, we can get involved with developing something better in our own mind by adding non-Reiki things and removing important elements of the class structure. When we get in the way it only starts diluting the strength and simplicity of the foolproof system entrusted to us from our Master and from Japan.

Hawayo Takata is quoted as saying, "If it isn't simple, it isn't Reiki. The power of the system lies in the pureness of the simplicity." When students would ask to take notes or have a class handout she would explain that she wanted the

Reiki information inside of them, not on a piece of paper somewhere. If they couldn't find the paper, they would feel they couldn't practice Reiki. After all, once you have a strong foundation you can't do Reiki wrong but you can always do it better. This is important to remember as we grow and travel on the Reiki pathway.

In Asian spiritual practices and martial arts, knowledge at times is divided into degrees. As the person integrates the lessons and develops the skills of one level, he or she progresses to the next level of understanding until they reach their highest potential. While many people are attracted to the most basic levels of training, intermediate and advanced levels may not be for everyone. Those who are called to become advanced students and practitioners often need to have a higher level of dedication and strength.

This can also be true for Reiki. A good number of people find all the healing they need in First or Second Degree training, while those of us that appear to connect on a deeper level can't seem to get enough Reiki, integrating it into all our daily activities. This usually indicates we are headed for the next step, which is to teach other people what we hold so dear and commit ourselves to Reiki Master training and living the life of Reiki.

First Degree Reiki

In First Degree Reiki training students receive 1) Four initiations, which is a ceremonial act that awakes the healing ability in the hands and allows it to flow in a precise manner 2) The history story of Usui Shiki Ryoho 3) Hand positions for treating self and other people 4) Five Spiritual Precepts (explained in the upcoming chapter "Reiki Precepts").

A 21-day cleansing process automatically begins after the training. This cleansing process is very individual depending on past history and current physical and emotional health.

As mentioned in the previous chapter when our energy is out of balance we can experience all sorts of illness and unrest. If we tend to be more of a giver or a receiver, instead of giving and receiving equally, the cleansing time often works to bring this into balance.

The physical body may clean itself by releasing toxins in the form of perspiration or through the urine and bowel movements. There have been a few times when students who had been on heavy medication for a while reported their tongue having a black film that went away after brushing. This was a way of pollutant release for their body. Students learn the value of applying Reiki energy to medications before taking them to help minimize their negative side-effects by naturally balancing the energy in the pills or capsules.

In First Degree Reiki class we learn to better handle our own energy and the energy of what affects us.

Self Treatment Is The Foundation Of Reiki Practice

First Degree Reiki is mostly about healing ourselves. In the beginning we may believe we are taking the training to heal someone else, our planet or whatever, but once the energy starts flowing the bottom line is: The more we heal ourselves, the more we heal our environment and additionally the more we have to share with other people. The world will not change until we do. When Reiki comes into our lives it expands us on all levels by healing us and everything around us.

Once we have completed Reiki initiations, it is impossible to attempt and heal anyone else without first having received healing ourselves. Why? Because the initiation process will open, balance and fine-tune our energy field allowing the energy to flow through us in a very precise manner like a funnel. It is then that the energy is continually present. This connection is never lost. The more we use it, the stronger it

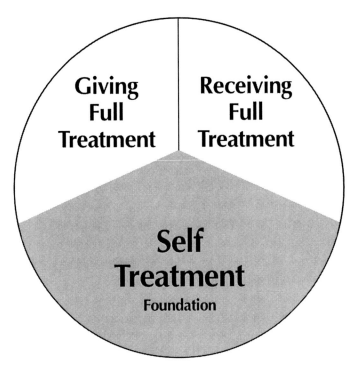

Reiki practitioners receive the most healing by starting and ending the day with full self-treatment then continuing to use Reiki in various ways throughout the day. The circle is complete by giving and receiving full hour treatments.

After being initiated into Reiki and all the exciting possibilities it offers, it is helpful to remember the benefits of balanced energy flowing in and out, out and in. To receive the most from this sacred practice we need to love ourselves enough to learn to enjoy the never-ending depths of the gift of self-treatment. This is the foundation of the practice of Reiki Natural Healing.

From this base we can easily expand upon giving full-hour treatments to others. The key is to appreciate ourselves enough to schedule to also receive these full treatments. Reiki and all of life is about giving and receiving in balanced harmony.

becomes. The energy flows through the practitioner before it reaches the person or thing we are applying our hands to. So, both parties receive the healing benefits simultaneously!

Through self-treatment all else can grow. Some find they need less sleep after receiving Reiki because they are replenishing their energy in a new way. Doing self-treatment in the evening relaxes the body, mind and spirit and encourages us to drift into a deep, restful night's sleep. It is also a delightful way to return to wakefulness, energize the body, and prepare to meet the day with a fresh perspective.

Doing this practice both in the morning and evening becomes a daily gift to ourselves and those with whom we contact. This habit can be the most valuable and nurturing maintenance plan available for our overall health and well-being. After a short while, practitioners become accustomed to living in the flow of life, watching as their daily activities become easier and more enjoyable.

Recalling the Reiki Precepts learned during First Degree training while giving self-treatment is a unique way to further support one's healing process. The combination of supportive energy with these simple guidelines for living is a potent combination for restoring health to the mind and emotions, which in turn benefits physical health.

In addition, practitioners may choose to put one or both of their Reiki-initiated hands on themselves as they go through their busy day. At work while in a meeting, or on the telephone, watching a movie or any time a hand is available is a good time to give your body more energy. We casually rest our hands on our chair, desks, computers and other things. Since Reiki provides an automatic flow upon contact why not Reiki yourself?

You will notice results from quickly relaxing emotions to healing a headache. Reiki is like a love bath for our personality and we all know that living in love is more fun and efficient than living in anxiety.

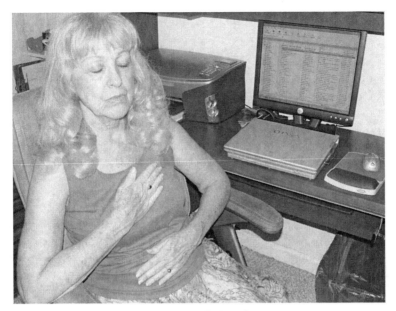

Take a Reiki break

A lady in First Degree training once told me, "First Degree Reiki is the gift of a dream come true."

Keep It Simple

During Reiki training it becomes very clear that the power of Reiki Natural Healing is in its simplicity and that it actually works better when we keep our mind out of it. Sometimes this is difficult for those of us in the Western World to comprehend. I often tell students the best way to describe Reiki to someone who asks what it is, is to offer to give them a mini-treatment. It's one of those things that can only be understood through experience.

Mrs. Takata, when asked what Reiki is, would answer, "It is God Power." How does it work? "Reiki on - Reiki off" was her answer. She was at times known, honored and loved for her directness and simplicity. She might offer further explanation by comparing the flow of Reiki to a broadcast from a radio transmitter, unseen, unheard until a receiver picks it up

and converts it into sound. In a similar way, she would explain
Reiki is always present, yet we are unaware of it until contact
is made through the training, after which it can be received
and converted into healing energy.

During her training Dr. Hayashi described to Mrs. Takata,
"Whenever I feel the contact, all I know is that I have
reached this great Universal Life Force, and it comes through
me to you—these," as he held up his hands, "are the elec-
trodes."

It is through this continual connection to a greater life
force that Reiki begins to work its healing influence from a
spiritual level.

Over the years, I've had the distinct honor and pleasure to
initiate hundreds of students into this sacred healing art and
witness how it works so uniquely with each individual to fulfill their personal healing needs.

Classes For Children

Reiki training is for everyone of all ages. Even though I
offer Keiki Reiki Classes (Keiki is the Hawaiian word for children) I actually have had more success teaching children of
all ages right along with the adults! They tend to act more
grown up, want to do as the adults do and seem to respect
and appreciate the confidence that is entrusted to them.
And adults learn from the clear mind and natural instincts of
children.

Unlike some Reiki Masters, the age of the child is not that
important to me. During my years of teaching it didn't take
long to discover that maturity, interest and connection to
Reiki can happen at any age. A fellow Reiki Master was assisting in the delivery of a baby. The mother was a Reiki practitioner and requested her child be initiated immediately after
birth. She explained that she knew whenever she touched
herself and other people that the automatic Reiki flow was

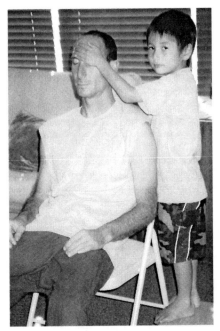

Children do well in Reiki classes along with the adults

producing healing results. Why wouldn't she want her baby to be giving herself Reiki when she placed her little hands on her body? Later when the child was ready she would be invited to attend formal Reiki training. The Reiki Master then sent a distant Reiki treatment to the unborn baby and received her energetic permission to initiate her into Reiki.

For many years the youngest child I had initiated was Britney at 7 years old. Then I had the honor to train 5 year old Kin, who is shown in the previous photo. A young couple came for training and their baby was expected in four months. As I was initiating the mother, I felt a need to also ask permission from the baby in her womb. I received a very clear positive response and knew immediately that the baby was a boy. Now the youngest child I have initiated is Kainalu Koa Wilson at five months in utero.

I have found it to be important for children to have an adult sponsor before being accepted for Reiki training—

Living a Life of Reiki

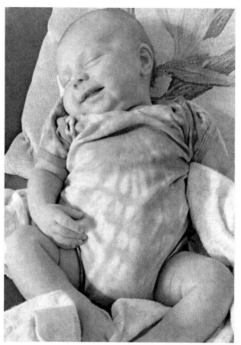

Kainalu Koa Wilson was initiated into Reiki while in utero

someone whom they respect and have a close connection with and one who has received Reiki initiations, preferably their parents. That way the child has a support person who will agree to assist in guiding the child's Reiki development. It is most helpful when they are able to practice self-treatments and full treatments together, along with regularly sharing the Reiki Precepts with each other. A "Reiki God Parent," if you will.

Before the training, I request a meeting to interview children. It is important that Reiki is something they want to do and not something another person wants for them. The child needs to understand the sacredness of Reiki, what it is about, and what will take place during the class. I ask that they earn at least half of the money for the training. It is especially sweet when children bring their money saving's container to class. They place their small hands around it and send it positive energy. Then proudly put it on the table in front of the four pictures of the Grand Masters, as a token of their commitment and the energy exchange that will be taking place.

Personally, I like to explain the pictures of the Reiki lineage bearers before class, sharing their names while observing how the child connects with their energy. I feel it is important for them to understand that we are grateful that Dr. Usui made an effort to create Reiki for us and we are happy the other three lineage bearers took good care of Reiki so we can have it today. Afterwards, I explain that Reiki is not something to be taken lightly—it is a very special gift and a responsibility comes along with it. The responsibility is called self-treatment and sharing treatments with other people, food, plants and animals, etc.

They love the idea that all they have to do to turn it on is to touch, as they are still open and exploring the world with their little hands. Children, like animals, are usually naturally receptive to what they know deep inside is good for them.

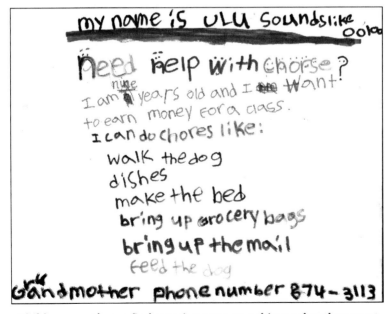

Children can always find creative ways to achieve what they want

Reiki Circle

From 1990 to 2006 on Tuesday evenings, I offered weekly Reiki healing circles on the island of Kauai, Hawaii. They provided an opportunity for local and visiting practitioners to experience group Reiki treatments as we came together and shared Reiki healing and our Reiki success stories with each other. At one time I had a gorgeous, loving, part German Shepard Reiki dog named Malia in my life. As practitioners parked their cars and strolled up the walkway to the house to attend our Reiki circle, she would happily run out to greet them and contently nestle her nose into the palm of their Reiki hand. At other times when guests arrived that were not Reiki initiated this didn't happen. As group Reiki energy started flowing, practitioners would chuckle to see Malia on the porch outside with all four legs in the air receiving her treatment.

Second Degree Reiki

Second Degree Reiki offers a review of First Degree training, one initiation, knowledge of the Reiki symbols and how to use them for mental, hands-on and distant treatments. This class is available to those who have faithfully practiced and received the benefits of self-treatment and have shared treatments with others.

The Second Degree student has matured to a place where they understand the practice on a deeper level. They have recognized the benefits of treatment and are ready to share more fully these benefits with other people.

A three-month minimum practice period for energy integration and comprehension is required before someone is eligible to take this training. My experience has been that when the student is ready and not before, Reiki will allow the next initiation to happen. It is a very personal process.

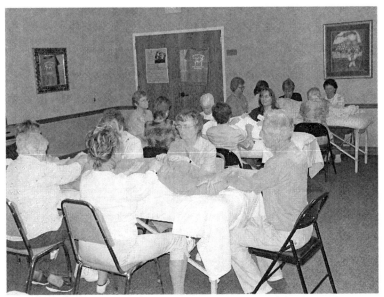

Reiki practitioners share Reiki healing in a Reiki circle

For many years I have taught classes away from Hawaii. There are times after a month long teaching tour that I return home to find Second Degree registrations and deposits from students who just completed their First Degree training during my tour. They are registering for my return visit in a few months.

It has been intriguing to witness the life span of these intentions. Some students are actually ready when the next class comes around, others have all sorts of things come up causing them to wait for a later training. Reiki clearly guides the way in divine timing.

In comparison, another student who had taken First Degree training from me while living on Kauai registered for a mainland U.S. Second Degree class twelve years later. My experience has shown that you will have no doubt when it is the right time for you. It is not something to think about you just know it is time for the next level of training.

When we are preparing to attend First Degree training we may wonder what we are getting into. No words can really explain what will be taking place in the classroom. There is simply an inner knowing present that I need to do this, I am not sure I understand it, but I simply need to take this training for whatever reason.

The idea that anyone can provide healing energy upon contact is not the way our society thinks in today's world. Then, after the training we are so excited because it works, it actually works!

Well, this level of trust and surrender is nothing compared to Second Degree training. Okay, I now understand that I can provide healing energy upon contact. Now, my Reiki Master is telling me I can provide it without contact. The person I'm giving a Reiki treatment to may be on the other side of the planet. How can this be possible?

Patiently and lovingly we explain that a hands-on treatment connects first with the physical body and then the energy may go to work with emotional healing. With distant treatments the practitioner is first connecting with the energetic body, which then may provide healing energy to the physical body. What a joy to discover this actually works too and even works better when the logical mind stays out of the way. Reiki continues to teach, if it isn't simple it isn't Reiki. What a relief and an exciting message to carry into other aspects of our lives.

Master Training

The path of the Reiki Master and the Reiki Master Candidate is never ending. It is a lifetime commitment, and some people believe, beyond lifetime. Master training is for those who wish to teach and live the life of Reiki. This final level of formal Reiki training is primarily dedication to self-development and to the sometimes demanding self-healing which is essential to understanding the healing process of our students and clients.

The Reiki Precepts that were learned in First Degree class start to take on a whole new meaning as they integrate more fully into all aspects of life. There is one initiation, the master kanji, and instructions for teaching and initiating others.

Mastership is about being there for your students and clients when needed. Being a Reiki Master is not a 9-to-5 job—it truly is a 24/7 commitment, all the while maintaining a healthy balance with our personal life.

Masters have inner strength for their students, teaching them by example to enjoy each moment of our precious lives and showing how we can hold a Reiki love vibration during times when we are faced with the challenges of rejection, denial and resistance to growth and change.

We learn when sensing those feelings of insecurity and struggle that we can be sure deep healing is taking place. Old energies that no longer serve us are being stirred up and released to make way for new more appropriate and conducive healing energies. Reiki is calling us to give up defensiveness and to rely on innate power; Reiki teaches us to find peace in any situation. In our classes we learn that it is not about always giving the answer but guiding and allowing the student to find their own answer.

It continues to amaze me even after years of teaching Reiki classes, if I'm not living in integrity with the Reiki Precepts, students in my class will clearly reflect back areas of my emotions that I need to bring back into alignment. As this action starts to push my emotional buttons, usually I can now (after many years of practice) recognize and appreciate that student as my teacher bringing this needed healing to my attention.

Being a Reiki Master means being prepared to stand outside our own healing when necessary to uphold the reverence of Reiki in our classroom. It is a lifetime of commitment to personal development and healing. Much practice time is recommended before considering this endeavor because we can't very well teach something we haven't personally experienced. A good example of this is how obvious it is when a Master is not living the Reiki Precepts. The healing energy just doesn't seem to be flowing effortlessly and smoothly. More about the Reiki Precepts will be explained in the next chapter.

One year is the very least amount of time after Second Degree before taking into consideration Master training. After acceptance as a Reiki Master Candidate and completing initial training of at least one year, the candidate is initiated as a Reiki Master and is ready to start teaching First and Second Degree students. At this stage, however, the new Master is still considered a "Master in training" for at least three years. After the initial three year period the new Master can meet with his or her Reiki Master and it will be known if he or she is ready to begin accepting Reiki Master Candidates for training.

One Master Candidate of mine didn't waste any time during her Master in training period, she actually taught a first degree student on the first day after her initiation ceremony!

When Masters begin to teach, it is a ride of ups and downs containing much personal healing, education, satisfaction, fun and rewards, along with various types of life-changing lessons along the way.

The personal restorative process can be quite enlightening as the Master receives all the initiations coming through them during their classes. Masters don't acquire more energy through their personal initiation process, they receive it by sharing initiations with their students. They start to notice that each student seems to bring similar energy to their own into class. Life takes on a whole new meaning as they share the joyful excitement and healing stories received from students, while at the same time recognizing them as their teacher.

Keeping it Pure

Because individuals have come for a Reiki hands-on healing class it is vitally important not to mix any other healing modalities or objects with our training. By keeping our classes clean we are honoring our students, ourselves and the reliability of the precious gift of Reiki Natural Healing. There are many ways to work with healing. Reiki is one of those ways and it is not to be mixed with another, even though we may think it will enhance the training or treatment. As the practitioner, the only thing that will add more healing to our Reiki treatment is receiving more Reiki ourselves. Some of Takata's student's have said that Mrs. Takata stressed this in her classes. She said to treat Reiki with the respect it deserves. And she also made it a point to tell her students to learn humility and heal the ego— that it blocks the way for pure healing to happen.

Another important consideration in keeping Reiki pure is for masters to be mindful of whom they teach. Friends and family members may have witnessed our positive changes and growth with Reiki during our Master training and be anxiously awaiting our initiation so we can share this new experience with them.

My belief is that complications (more times than not) arise when we initiate our family members into Reiki. It is difficult to respect someone as your Reiki Master after sharing years of various types of playful intimate relationship. You may, first of all, be their Mommy, so where does that leave the respect and sacredness for their Reiki Master? Memories of us as Auntie or Uncle or Mom or Dad can get in the way of holding reverence and respect for us as their Reiki Master. It just seems too confusing for most people, especially children.

The role of a Reiki Master is to be available when called upon to nurture the seed of Reiki that was planted with the sacred initiations. It is tricky to hold a friendship or family relationship and also be available to continually teach and guide the loved one with pure Reiki energy along their healing path.

Remember, we don't give our Reiki away. A money energy exchange for Masters providing service of training and full-hour treatments is a valuable part of the healing process, for ourselves as well as the person with whom we are sharing the healing energy.

Masters surrender and trust on a new level when they become full-time Reiki Masters. Each aspect of the system continues to deepen, including our relationship with money. We gain understanding on deeper and deeper levels how money is nothing more than flowing energy, continually moving in and out—out and in, creating one harmonious flow to sustain us. Why would it not work like everything else in our universe? Knowing without a doubt that the only thing slowing down or stopping its flow are thoughts and feelings that create blocked energy around it.

Usui Shiki Ryoho teaches not to promote poverty consciousness. Our class fees have been established for many important healing reasons. The same price in U.S. dollars is charged no matter where we teach in the world. It is such a gratifying validation when you witness a student, who struggled to acquire the funds for First Degree, work smoothly with this in and out energy of life and be able to easily provide the money for Second Degree and Master Training.

I am constantly reminded of that old proverb: "Which is better? To give someone a fish and let them eat for one day, or teach them how to fish to provide nourishment for a lifetime?"

A Year in the Life of a Reiki Master Candidate

By Diane Larson, Reiki Master

My year of Reiki Master training is something hard for me to put into words. I guess to say what didn't come up for me would be more appropriate. Many things I thought I knew took on a whole new meaning. Lessons I needed to learn came to the forefront. Aspects and old belief systems needed to be examined and rearranged. In essence I became a new me!

When I began to trust Reiki on every level a sense of liberation swept over me. To feel this free was something that was unfamiliar to me, yet inherently I knew was my birthright.

To live this dance with Reiki has brought me unimaginable joy. Not to say that I don't occasionally fall back into my, not so good for me ways, but with Reiki by my side I feel like I found my best friend! I'd like to share with you just as I finished that last sentence a rainbow appeared for just a few seconds over the ocean in Hana.

I have learned that Reiki will provide whatever I need as long as I dedicate and commit myself to it whole heartily. To exude this faith and belief that Reiki will consistently be there for me is profound beyond words.

To have been blessed with the most impeccable Reiki Master, Shalandra Abbey, to guide and illuminate my path is an incredible honor. Shalandra lives and breathes Reiki and if I can one day hold a candle to her, it would be all I could hope for.

Without the Grand Masters of Reiki I wouldn't be writing this announcement. Their energy has given me strength when I was being the most challenged. Their words of wisdom and belief in me has been a powerful force. Thank you Dr. Usui, Dr. Hayashi, Mrs. Takata and Ms. Furumoto for choosing me to be a Reiki Master!

Diane Larson is a full-time Reiki Master on the island of Maui, Hawaii. www.MauiIslandReiki.com

The Path Of Mastery

1. Usui Shiki Ryoho (Usui System of Reiki) is a way of life for its masters. There is honor and respect that masters remain students and not creators of the system. Appreciation for the simplicity and power of Reiki grows as we grow.

2. Masters agree to use the form as it is cared for by the current lineage bearer Phyllis Lei Furumoto, honoring that she has been chosen to be the bearer of this lineage. She carries the seed of Usui Shiki Ryoho passed from one generation to another, and it is her responsibility to see that the seed is passed on without distortion.

3. "Surrender" to the flow of the guidance of the Reiki energy becomes an exciting way to trust life without the need to know why. However, there is the continual awareness that we are partners with Reiki. We don't just turn over our lives. We use our power of choice.

4. The Reiki Alliance is a voluntary body of masters who come together through a common commitment and desire for a Reiki Master Community.

5. Masters and Master Candidates have a lifelong commitment to each other. Candidates receive support on their teaching journey. They mature as a team in mutual respect.

6. Masters are encouraged to explore areas in their communities where they feel drawn to work with Reiki. Documentation of the results is important for future introduction of Reiki.

7. Acceptance, understanding and respect of other Reiki masters and students are important. By recognizing what is shared in common and acknowledging differences, we grow with the flow of the life force energy and create a better world.

As we integrate Reiki into our various health care systems, continuing education credit is helpful for students of Reiki Natural Healing. My classes are approved to provide CE credit for nurses and massage therapists.

The more we use Reiki, the more energy can pour through us. Reiki Training is similar to a lifetime of ongoing Reiki treatments and more. A student once said: "Reiki is like a kiss. It needs to be shared to be fully enjoyed."

The word Reiki in Japanese consists of two parts. The top is "Rei" and the bottom is "Ki" meaning Universal Energy.

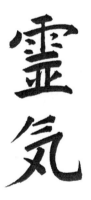

When I speak of my work, what I'm referring to is the sacred profession of Reiki.

An important step on the Reiki journey—the
Precepts of Reiki help us to heal our thoughts.
What lessons do they hold for you?

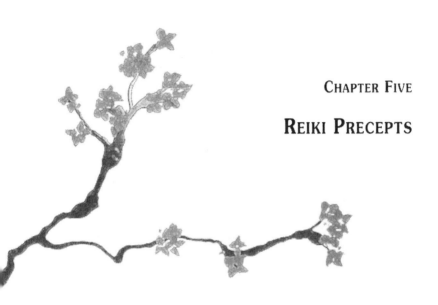

CHAPTER FIVE

REIKI PRECEPTS

Spiritual Precepts of Reiki

Just for today, do not worry.
Just for today, do not anger.
Honor your parents, teachers, and elders.
Earn your living honestly.
Show gratitude to every living thing.

By Dr. Mikao Usui, Founder of Reiki Natural Healing

D r. Mikao Usui, the first Reiki Grand Master, received in meditation and then further developed the five Reiki Precepts after he decided to leave the Beggars Quarters of Kyoto where he first introduced Reiki in Japan.

He had gone there to start sharing Reiki healing, thinking it was where it was most needed. During his stay Dr. Usui became aware of some important aspects of human nature. He had begun these Reiki healing treatments in the hope of providing beggars an opportunity to become integrated into the structure of society. When several tried and failed at shouldering the responsibilities of everyday life in regular society, he began to recognize the importance of a person's participation in their own life healing process.

His realization that a person needs to want and then ask for a change or healing to make a real difference in their life is as true today as it was in those days. If the help of another person is involved in the process of making changes or healing, there also needs to be an exchange of energy for the time, effort and expenses of the person helping. By just giving away Reiki healing, Usui recognized he had actually further impressed the pattern of begging and poverty in many of them.

He saw the need for people to give back for what they receive in order to maintain a sense of balance and not carry around a feeling of indebtedness. Making an appropriate offering for a healing treatment empowers the self and develops positive self-worth. It is not the job of anyone to try and help where it is not wanted.

Dr. Usui also learned the importance of non-attachment to the results of his treatments. It is possible that some of the beggars needed to live out their lives in the Beggars Quarter in order to learn certain lessons. Who was he to judge this as right or wrong? The same non-judgment applies to disease.

Every experience in life is an opportunity for us to learn and grow. Sometimes the initiation for this learning comes from a soul level and is buried deep in the unconscious self. A person might create a disease on a subconscious level to enable them to learn particular lessons, or perhaps, even to die in a certain manner. As practitioners we don't invade this highly personal space by projecting our belief about the reason for someone's illness. Whatever the learning is, it is up to the individual to navigate his or her own path. The role of the practitioner is simply to allow the Reiki energy to flow and support the healing process.

This truth became very clear to Usui as he recognized that it was not his job to use his incredible gift to heal the world as he had originally seen it, but indeed to show people how they might help themselves heal their own lives in a broader way. In this way, the world would then heal itself. It was during this time that he understood people need guidelines to help them grow in understanding, and that it was his role to assist them to shoulder greater responsibility for their own life situations.

Dr. Usui realized that he had healed the physical body of symptoms but had not taught appreciation for life nor for a new way of living. Shortly afterwards he received the powerful Reiki Precepts. Reiki practitioners strive to live these Precepts each day, which helps heal the mind and emotions. By doing so, they find more respect for themselves, the world and all those around them.

The five Precepts that Usui taught emanate naturally from a person who experiences his or her balanced flow of healing. Starting immediately to live these Reiki Precepts helps put a person in that flow, because what we think and how we feel truly determine what we are.

There are many ways to interpret the Precepts. These ways change and evolve as we grow in our spiritual development. Throughout the day the Precepts become reminders to us and help us to stay in alignment with our own best qualities and those of our environment.

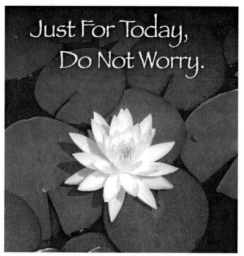

Precept number one

Just for today, do not worry

To worry is to forget that there is a divine or universal purpose in everything. By doing self-treatment we are truly in close touch with the guidance of the energy of life. We start to understand that there isn't anything more important than what is happening right now. This helps us to live each day to the best of our ability. There is a natural awareness that we have done our part and the rest is up to our source. Worry is a thought pattern that results from a feeling of separateness, of being disconnected from the wholeness of life. When we remember that each person, including ourselves, does the best we can in each of life's situations in accordance with the knowledge or wisdom we have at any given moment we begin to realize that to worry is futile and most of what we worry about never happens anyway. We learn to change the emotion of worry to one of gratitude and all becomes well with each precious moment. Just for today, do not worry.

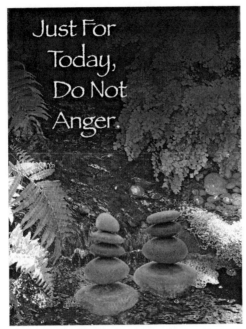

Precept number two

Just for today, do not anger

To anger is to judge and desire control; we want things to be the way we think is the right way. We don't recognize that on some level there is no right way, it is an individual truth for each of us. Anger becomes a defense mechanism when we are not empowered. We quickly become a victim and want to fight back from a helpless feeling of being out of control. We have allowed the ego to direct our life while ignoring our inner guidance that would guide us to a natural and harmonious flow. When our expectations are not met—perhaps because someone or even ourselves didn't live up to our needs and desires—often the result is anger. When our feelings are not coming from the energy of unconditional love, we can learn to let them go and feel gratitude for having been given an opportunity for growth. Just for today, do not anger.

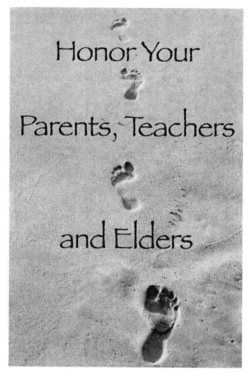

Honor Your Parents, Teachers and Elders

Precept number three

Honor your parents, teachers, and elders

To live in gratitude for those who have made major differences in our life is to live in abundance. If we can truthfully look at uncomfortable feelings about someone and acknowledge them as emotional energy blocks within ourselves (which affect the health of our body, mind and spirit) we can move forward with healing them much more rapidly. Our parents are usually the first and last people we have contact with, so there may be healing needed with them. Once more we can practice the attitude of gratitude. When we are constantly grateful for what we have received and for what we know and trust, our needs continue to be provided for. Acknowledging everyone we met in life as our teacher while making a conscious effort to connect more with the elders offers more possibilities for gratitude, peace and joy. Honor your parents, teachers, and elders.

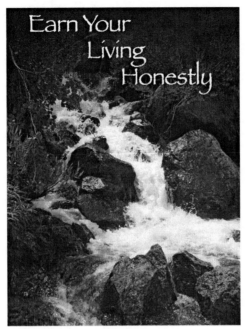

Precept number four

Earn your living honestly

Of great importance for a harmonious life flow is honesty in dealing with one's self. To be honest with oneself is to face the truth in all things. When we are honest with our self, we project honesty onto others and in turn only the energy of honesty will return to us. It then becomes easy to "do unto others, as we would have others do unto us." Giving and receiving in balance keeps the energy of health and happiness moving in the Universal flow. When we earn our living honestly we are being truthful to our self, and we help create peace and harmony in our life and our world. Earn your living honestly.

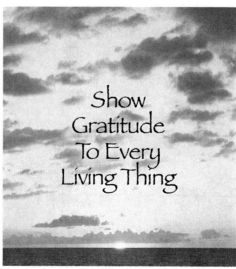

Precept number five

Show gratitude to every living thing

Every living thing was created for a divine purpose and from the same source. All forms of matter vibrate at different energy levels, yet they are all interconnected because there are no solid barriers between them. Thus, when we accept all of the various aspects of ourselves it affects all others. Likewise, when we accept others, we feel the reflection in ourselves. Any positive energy, whether directed at others or ourselves, helps to heal the whole planet. Each person, animal, plant, and mineral is included in the whole. Respecting all life forms as our brothers and sisters is another way to stay connected to the flow of life and to bring more health, love and abundance to us all. To show love and respect to all is to love and respect our mother earth and our selves. When we understand that all forms of life are interdependent we more naturally can bring the attitude of gratitude to all we come in contact with. Show gratitude to every living thing.

I encourage you to pay attention to these Precepts as you go through the day. How many times do you block your natural flow of healthy energy with the emotions of worry and anger? It can be a surprising revelation and a great way to start decreasing some of the illness in our world today.

Reiki Is A Spiritual Discipline

Reiki Natural Healing is a spiritual discipline practiced by people from many different religions or none at all. For me feeling Reiki energy is like seeing a brightly colored rainbow and experiencing it profoundly within my heart.

Reiki is love energy, and a person normally experiences Reiki feeling that deep spiritual inner love connection with themselves and all that exists. It is a truly special and powerful opportunity to contemplate the Reiki Precepts during Reiki treatments for one's self.

My recommendation is to give yourself the gift of self-treatment as soon as you open your eyes in the morning and the last thing before falling asleep at night. Anytime during the day that you can place a hand on yourself is a good time for Reiki.

In the morning during self-treatment is a good time to think about what plans you have for the day. Ask yourself, "What situations have the possibility of bringing up the emotions of Worry—Anger—Honoring my parents, teachers and elders—Earning my living honestly—Showing gratitude to every living thing? How can I live the energy of the Precepts during this day?"

At night it is often encouraging, sometimes a little discouraging, to review how well you did applying the Precepts to your day's life experiences.

Were you able to recall the details of the day without the slightest emotion of worry or anger? If you started to worry, did you immediately use our first Reiki Precept and the attitude of gratitude to transmute that feeling to a more fruitful energy?

How did you handle the anger when it started to surface in an instance when the person, who didn't understand your words, lashed out at you? Knowing that when we fly into a rage we always make a bad landing.

Could you feel love from your heart going to their heart to assist the energy to balance and understanding to come forth? Or, was your anger present from trying to control or judge that person?

How did you honor that new cashier at the department store who made you late for your next appointment? Did you show him gratitude for being your spiritual teacher and no longer allowing you to blindly rush through the day, for slowing you down and providing the opportunity for understanding the all-important lessons of patience and compassion? Remember we awaken in others the same attitude of mind we hold toward them.

Some students think that it is too difficult to work with all the Precepts in the beginning, so they prefer focusing on one at a time until they are ready to graduate to the next. Working with the Precepts is a healing cycle. Once we sense we have finally gotten it and are doing well with a certain Precept, life has fun testing us, urging us to move forward to the next level of understanding and healing with it. There is no end to the lessons the Reiki Precepts provide us.

The exciting part is how much freer and healthier we become as we allow them to assist us to be happier people. It is sad to consider the vast amount of people in our world today that are sick because of the energetic effects of worry or anger. The Reiki Precepts show us how to recognize and then clear away that blocked energy in order to tap into more positive and creative energies.

Webster's Collegiate Dictionary explains these words for us.

Worry – to afflict with mental distress or agitation: make anxious.

Anger – a strong emotion induced by intense displeasure.

Honor – a showing of respect.

Earn – to receive a return for effort.

Gratitude – the state of being grateful.

What do these words mean for you in your life? Are you allowing your energy around these emotions to flow in harmony and balance? If not—why not? Start today making an effort to heal emotional issues that no longer serve you. The benefits are well worth the endeavor.

At our annual International Reiki Alliance conferences there are many different languages represented. It can be a powerful moment when a representative from each shares the Precepts in the language of their country. I remember one year in Germany there were 27 languages spoken, creating really yummy healing from our international Reiki Precept energy.

You too can heal with your words in so many different ways. Recently someone brought to my attention that they find it interesting to note that in the Hawaiian language, there are no swear words. This is probably because of the old Hawaiian saying, "Words can heal, or words can kill." This wise adage holds a valuable lesson.

A few years ago, a student of mine named Noboru attended my First Degree class. It was an honor indeed to initiate him into Reiki. The first day of class I explained the Reiki Precepts. The second day when he returned to class he had written them in Japanese on rice paper for the other eleven students and myself. Thanks to Noboru's gift and thoughtfulness, I share those here with you.

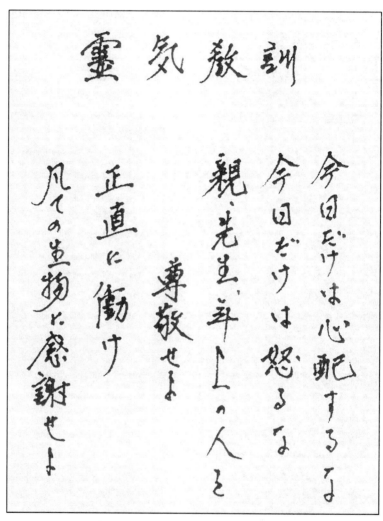

霊 気 敎 訓

今日だけは心配するな

今日だけは怒るな

親、先生、年上の人を

尊敬せよ

正直に働け

凡ての生物に感謝せよ

Reiki Precepts hand written in Japanese

Giving and receiving money in balance is important to our health. See how the flow of energy in our lives directly affects the flow of money, and how Reiki can lead to unlimited abundance.

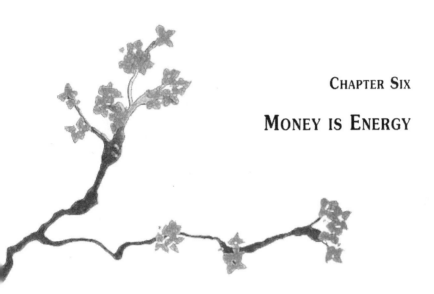

CHAPTER SIX

MONEY IS ENERGY

J ust as the emotions of worry and anger cause a multitude of illnesses in our world today, so it is with money.

If we look back in time to its creation, money was merely the next step after the barter system. We created money to use as a form of energy exchange. When a person didn't have fruit to exchange for vegetables or an item of equal value, they gave a promissory note. So it became the custom that as individuals extended and gave of their energy, they received money in exchange. The more we use Reiki energy and stay connected to our source of creation, the more clarity we receive around the energy of money.

In today's world it seems the majority of things we do, even our reputation, can be formed as a result of money. Often when the money word is uttered, or even when we see a picture of it, it sends out an incredibly high charge of energy and is interpreted in a way that depends on where we are with our relationship to it.

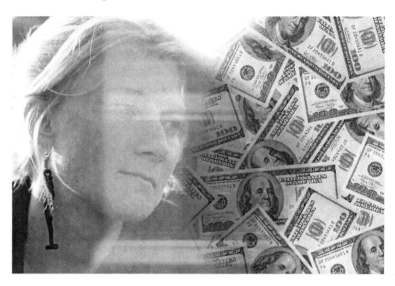

Blocked Energy Stops The Flow Of Money

Young children, and even babies in the womb, exposed to the energy of anxiety and anguish around money can become programmed with negative beliefs around money. Pregnant women are recognizing the value of playing soothing music for their unborn child, and yet may not recognize that the child is hearing conversations as well. For many couples, knowing a new baby is on its way may represent added financial obligations and they don't realize their unborn child is tuning into sometimes frustrating conversations around it. For instance, a couple expecting a baby may have discussions filled with concern and anxiety about their ability to adequately support their child.

The young child learns to identify money as something important to have. They are encouraged to stash away precious coins in piggy banks, or they may have a bank savings account. As they grow older they are told that they must save money to buy this or that thing considered a need or to satisfy a desire for material things.

An unhealthy relationship prevails in our culture and is reinforced by the media. Some religions today still teach us that to serve ourselves is selfish. Many people are taught to believe that providing only for basic necessities is enough and to become rich is wrong. Yet, some of our most affluent institutions are religious in nature. Our social order teaches that money has to be earned by hard work—even at a job we dislike. Struggling for money has become a way of life. Worries and anxiety over what appears to be an insufficient money source causes emotional energy blocks within our being, and this situation creates a deterrent to the energetic flow of money trying to come to us.

The more Reiki teaches us to understand energy, the clearer the nature of these imbalances become to us. For existence to be harmonious, an even balanced flow of, "in and out—out and in" exchange of energy, is necessary in all areas of life.

Money is energy and our thought forms can create a blockage to its flow into our wallets and bank accounts. It is a process similar to the natural flow of rainwater in the mountains flowing down the streams into a vast ocean. When blockages such as rocks and trees get in the way, the flow slows down. If they are removed the water flows at a swifter pace.

Once we begin to experience Reiki Natural Healing and recognize how we are connected to all of life, we start to identify energy blocks all around us.

What are energy blocks? Anything that is stopping that flow of the unlimited abundance that is our birthright is considered an energy block.

What We Envision In Our Minds Becomes Our World

Our brain operates like a computer software program. Each time we utter the words, "I don't have the money" (for this or that), we produce it in our database and create all sorts of events to keep it from coming to us, because our program is "I don't have money." It is astounding to discover that by simply changing our thoughts around money, we can create it in unlimited abundance. Our use of Reiki energy supports the process and keeps the money energy clear and flowing. We learn to continually generate and maintain clean energy about money.

What is constantly amazing about it is: We don't even need to know where the money is coming from; we just need to know for sure that it will be there when needed and wanted.

Sometimes our abundance doesn't necessarily come in the form of actual money, but in the form of what we envisioned buying with that money. As an example, the neighbor down the street all of a sudden is moving and wants to gift us with that new sofa we truly love and have been admiring during every visit. We acquire what we have wished for and it is delivered right to us!

It is so vitally important that we stay open to the brilliant and unlimited possibilities of life. When we are open on all levels to receive abundance, the flow of Reiki energy can bring us something even more magnificent than we imagined.

Maintain Connection To The Divine Flow

Reiki practitioners have great tools for creating boundless opulence in all areas of their lives. Working with healing energy through self-treatment, treatments with other people, and the Reiki Precepts on a daily basis maintains our connection to the divine flow. It is a universal law that everything flows in and out in balance. If we have been giving a lot out, it is only a matter of time before the flow returns to us as we learn to receive. Reiki helps a person relax deeply and quiet the mind, which of course is the first step to bring money and other forms of riches into our life.

The Reiki Precepts also support us to calm and heal the emotions. If you feel yourself doubting and questioning; that is what I have been referring to as creating blocked energy to keep it from coming into you. Let it go! It is certainly worth a try.

Surrender to the fact that all things just may be possible when your mind gets out of the way. Instead of doubting, feel yourself already having what you want and do not try to control the timing or way it will come to you. Once you put the energy of the request into motion, it will flow back to you at the perfect time, even though you may think there was a mistake in the timing, there really wasn't. The universal life force energy doesn't make mistakes.

Triumph Over The Fear Of Money

After Reiki initiations, the power of the universe clearly guides those who will follow.

My first major lesson in triumphing over the fear of money came at an early period in my Reiki life. In 1988, I was guided to leave the IBM Corporation in Coral Gables, Florida and move to Hawaii to live the life of a Reiki Master. It was hard for me to even think of telling my family and colleagues. Dreams of large, blue, beautiful ocean waves, sandy beaches and coconut trees came to me at night, and a psychic shared with me, "A big move is coming for you and you are going to live in a location that starts with the letter H."

"Why now?" I thought. At a time when I had a good career and was making a terrific income with a tremendous benefits package? Life was good. Why mess it up?

When I finally had the courage to take the big step, announcing it to my manager and co-workers was unbelievably scary. Most everyone figured I was going through a midlife crisis and gently suggested that I needed to wait a while longer because I only had a few more years before receiving the vested rights package and retirement benefits.

It is really humorous now (it certainly wasn't then) as I look back on my first few years living on the island of Kauai—struggling to hold on to money and to have at least some savings in the bank account.

Towards the end of my money reserve, real fear set in. But once the money was consumed there was an unexpected feeling of relief; it was as if a heavy burden had been lifted off my back. I could now truly support Reiki as long as it supported me. What a joy it was to discover that it would. In no uncertain terms, it would!

A Reiki Master's Job Description Is To Teach Reiki

Reiki Natural Healing had become the best teacher and employer I ever had. It wasn't easy because I had an entirely new way of life to learn. In this new life it was mandatory to leave old habits and belief systems behind. The warm familiar ones that had been my support system for most of my life had to go. Mainly using my analytical mind was no longer appropriate.

The Reiki Precepts teach us, "Just for today do not worry." Not about anything, including money. What a delight it was, to realize all that I ever need will always be there waiting for me, if I just stay out of the way. Seldom do I know how these needs will be met and at times they seem to arrive at the very last minute, but after twenty years of practicing Reiki I can tell you the needs never arrive late. If there seems to be a delay, check in with yourself for energy blocks in your thought forms. Once those are cleared, the money is able to start flowing again. At times it is not easy, but it is a straightforward process that always works.

The benefits package of a Reiki Master is quite different than most. Vacations, like money, come at the most unexpected times and locations. I find myself traveling to places I felt I couldn't afford or have the time for while working in the corporate world. Who would have thought I would have a job where I could do my work any place in the world my heart desires? There's no traditional job description with Reiki either and it can be a challenging proposition learning to trust and give in to the flow of the energy's guidance.

In my Reiki life I have passed test after test of challenges. At times it has been like walking off a high cliff to find I could fly with the energy of life—all the while continuing to find deeper levels of understanding in the importance of keeping my limited mind out of the way. Words cannot explain the sheer joy I have found experiencing these thrilling leaps of faith.

I have tasted what it is like to become one with and supported by all of life. The long-term benefits to being a Reiki Master include no terminations or lay-offs. When we learn to get out of the way of ourselves, we see clearly how life can be healthy and rewarding so there is no desire to quit.

Cash For My New Car

After several years of trusting and proving that money would come to cover my needs and wants, I decided it was time for a new car. For me, a used car wasn't an option. It needed to be and smell brand spanking new and, since the manifestation juices were flowing, why not add to the request that it be a cash purchase?

When it didn't come to pass in the expected timeframe it

made me wonder if just possibly I had asked for too much. Just thinking in these terms caused the vision to fade away.

Later, after I quit thinking about it, a sizable burst of money energy hit my Reiki practice. Each time I picked up the phone someone was requesting Reiki speaking engagements, treatments and training. I no longer had a savings account since the corporate money was gone, and I wondered why a great influx of income was occurring at this time. What was I to do with this financial over abundance that was so graciously coming to me?

For the previous ten years my lesson had been to create an even flow of money coming in and out, out and in. It was a fun, carefree way to live. At this point in my life I didn't want a savings account somewhere to block this magnificent flow. The only thing to do was send distant Reiki to the situation, sit in front of the pictures of the Reiki Grand Masters and simply ask, "Why is all this money coming to me at this time—what is it to be used for?" It was as if all four Grand Masters told me at the same time in no uncertain terms, "Well you said you wanted a new car!"

Months had passed since thinking about it, and so it truly caught me by surprise. Following a thrilling synchronicity of events I found myself on a teaching tour on the mainland U.S. and was guided to the perfect dealer with a good price for the car I wanted.

That was unexpected too; I only looked at one model and color of car, and just knew there was no need to look further. After all, a gold color car with champagne interior was perfect for the energy I was carrying. The cost was much less than in Hawaii, even after paying shipping expenses. A smile continues to appear on my face whenever I remember how, in my corporate life, I never felt I could afford to pay cash for an automobile. Talk about feeling like an empowered Reiki Master! Handing that money to the dealer was an extraordinarily rewarding experience that I shall never forget.

The Flow Of Energy Pays The Rent

There had been a powerfully intense time several years before that when Reiki and the energy of money taught me another important and unforgettable lesson around the issue of trust in the divine flow.

After returning from a three month teaching tour in Australia, I was guided to rent a home much more expensive than usual for me. It was simply the only house that felt right at the time and it was located on the beautiful north shore of Kauai, where I hadn't lived before. I had only dreamt how laid back and relaxing life must be on the tropical north shore. It was out of the blue because it was quite a distance away from the central location of my clients who came for treatments before the Australian sojourn.

Not long after being in the home I met an amazing man. We enjoyed each other's company so much and were together almost all the time, so we came to a decision to share the same home. It was a beautiful, fun relationship for several months and then it was time to separate. He had been paying the rent and I hadn't fully stepped into giving treatments and training again after returning from Australia.

It was the middle of the month when we parted and soon the realization came that I didn't have the money for the rent that was due in a few days. Like most any Reiki Master would do, I sat down and sent a distant Reiki treatment to the situation—asking the energy for assistance in this state of affairs, then waited for the answer to come.

A week passed with little action and no monetary manifestation, and only a few days left before the first of the month when the rent was due. Opening the mail that day there was an invitation for a birthday party cruise on the Mexican

Rivera, a 100th birthday party celebration for a beautiful
healer from Sedona. My inner knowing was telling me to send
the deposit now to attend. I looked up in the air saying, "wait
a minute, I don't have the money for the rent and the energy
is guiding me to send in this deposit."

Well, of course, before I knew what happened a check
went in the mail to accept the invitation, still not knowing
where the rent money would come from. It seemed to be
another big test in the making regarding trust and surrender,
which of course was exactly the catalyst for the energy of
money to flow back to me.

Soon after mailing the deposit, which took most of the
funds left, the phone rang. It was Donna and Robert who told
me, "It is time for us to move to Arkansas and our house has-
n't sold. We were wondering if you would be interested in
caretaking it for us until it sells. We are sure the Reiki energy
will help draw the perfect buyer to our home."

Within a matter of days I had moved back to the central
part of the island into a gorgeous home on the rim of the
Wailua River, one of the most sacred rivers in all of Hawaii,
and was enjoying the relaxing pleasure of the heated indoor
swimming pool while looking at the moon above me through
the skylight.

Of course it came with the added benefit of the perfect
setting for Reiki treatments and initiations. As students sat in
chairs in the private backyard near the ridge of the ravine,
they were viewing a majestic tropical paradise as they listened
to the birds singing to the healing music of the waterfalls
below.

Allow The Energy To Flow Back To You

When our money supply is low we have a tendency to
hold on to it, which of course is blocking its natural flow.
There was a time when I realized I was down to my last $100

bill. Panic started to set in so I quickly said the Reiki Precepts as I filled myself and the bill with healing energy. During this process I saw myself taking the carefully folded and protected $100 bill and exchanging it for one dollar bills. Returning home with the money, the message was to sit in the middle of my bed and toss the one hundred pieces of paper up in the air freely, while watching them return back down to me.

Try this sometime. It isn't as silly or as easy a thing to do as it sounds. It is well worth the effort. The message that came to me while I was doing it was, "This is the only way it can return to you." When we allow the energy of life to freely take its natural course and refrain from getting in the way of the divine flow, the process will be organically supported.

The moral of these stories is: Money is energy and once we can become friends with it and dance joyfully with its energy only goodness can follow. The boogey men are chased away. As we free ourselves of the blocked, unhealthy energy, we can use the new energy in more fun and productive ways. We discover that when we love what we do, we feel as if we will never have to work another day in our life. A non-Reiki book that can help to deepen understanding around the energy of money and is fun reading material is Lynn Grabhorn's book, *Excuse Me Your Life Is Waiting*. The information in her book, combined with Reiki energy, is a dynamic duo to keep the money energy alive and well.

Watching the dynamics around money when it comes to Reiki treatments and training can be deeply revealing. Giving money is a sacred act and is a means for the student to find their practice. It is a part of the spiritual path and part of the form of Usui Shiki Ryoho (Usui System of Reiki). The uniqueness and beauty of the healing power of this exchange for treatments is difficult to explain in limited words.

Reiki clients and practitioners I know agree there simply is not enough money available in the world to pay for the healing received while experiencing Reiki treatments. As money is exchanged, there are many different healings taking place in body, mind and spirit for both the giver and receiver.

Public Practice

The process that takes place when a student feels they are ready for public practice reminds me of First Degree training, where we are taught that when we give Reiki Natural Healing to someone else, we also receive it ourselves. The energy flows through us, we benefit. Total balance of giving and receiving takes place. A Reiki treatment is a form of service to others and in so doing it is a form of service to ourselves. That's the Reiki Way!

When a public practice is opened there are expenses involved. Actually the expenses begin with Reiki training, then a professional space, a Reiki table, and supplies for client and practitioner to be comfortable during treatment.

The treatment fee also needs to be established. This usually brings up all kinds of money issues to be healed for the practitioner and the clients they draw to them. What is a fair fee to charge? What if the client has expectations and isn't happy with what they receive during the treatment? Is the amount adequate for my time and expense; is it fair to the client and to Reiki? Is it honoring all concerned?

The emotions that go through the practitioner's mind when they are handed payment for the first treatment clearly shows where they are in their process of healing around the issue of money. Learning to respond to clients that want your time for no fee, or for an exchange of energy, can bring up all sorts of different kinds of hidden agendas to be healed for the participants.

By charging for our service, we don't leave someone in an owing position, making it uncomfortable for them to ask us for more treatments. Nor do we take away their dignity by thinking they can't afford to pay for their treatment.

At the same time, we are honoring ourselves by valuing our precious training, expenses and time extended. The more we respect ourselves, our clients and Reiki Natural Healing, the more self-esteem and confidence we have to offer, and the more professional service we provide.

Deeper Levels Of Healing Insecurity

Similarly, when masters start teaching Reiki, levels of insecurities can come to the surface for healing. A good example of this was given by our third Grand Master Hawayo Takata when her master Dr. Hayashi warned her by saying, "Whenever you become a master, never do it for free, because they will never use it, because it was free. It then has no value."

Mrs. Takata said, "I asked my teacher: 'Dr. Hayashi, will you permit and consent that I have one class free? And that is for all the people that have helped me through this year of sorrow and my sickness.' I said, I would like to teach them and give them a free lesson in Reiki so that they could benefit."

Her master replied, "Now that you are well, you can return your gratitude by giving them treatment when they need it, but not to say I'll hold a class for you."

With this understanding Mrs. Takata said, "Well I have to try. And so the first people that I gave free lessons were my best friend and relatives. They were my in-laws. All my in-laws had free lessons, and then my neighbors. And then when my two sisters came, I said, 'Wait, wait. I'm not going to teach you yet.' So, my sisters were kind of upset and said, 'Well we heard from your neighbors and in-laws that you taught them something really wonderful.'" Mrs. Takata replied, "At the moment, I will say no."

One day as Mrs. Takata was hanging her laundry her

neighbor came and said, "My daughter didn't go to school today because she has a little stomach ache. And so I brought her to you."

When Mrs. Takata asked why she had not given her a Reiki treatment she said, "You are the expert that lives next to me. So, it's easier to bring her to you than do it myself because I know she'll get well."

After this happened a few more times, Mrs. Takata went in her house and cried and looked towards Japan. She bowed her head to Dr. Hayashi and Dr. Usui and said, "Forgive me for being wrong. I did not help any person because they did not accept this gratefully and spiritually, because they didn't spend a penny."

After three months Hawayo Takata's sisters came again to ask for Reiki. She told them there is a fee for learning Reiki. Her sister said she needed to go home and talk with her husband about it. The husband said, "If you ask her for the Reiki then you should pay her for it." And so Takata taught her sisters Reiki. Later her sister returned to apologize for complaining about paying for her Reiki.

"I now know why you charged me because you wanted me to be a good practitioner. I do not have any more medicine bills and doctor bills, I don't have to go to the hospital every time I have a cold or every time I'm asthmatic, or every time bronchitis comes or my stomach aches. I appreciate it so much and will make good use of it."

And she did. She became a very successful business woman and used Reiki on her three children. She told Takata, "It was the cheapest investment I've made." And whenever she saw her sister she would offer to give her Reiki treatments because of her gratitude.

Mrs. Takata commented that none of the people she had given free Reiki training to were using it nor taking advantage of its many benefits. She hadn't been fair to her students or to herself. Her master was absolutely right when he warned her about giving Reiki away. Teaching people Reiki who do not use it is not going to change the world. The energy of money becomes an important part of the healing process for all parties concerned.

This was unmistakably proven to me when a young lady called and was interested in training and told me she didn't have the money for the class. Her husband had made his transition and she had expenses of three small children.

I suggested she find a pretty envelope and write the words "Reiki Training" on it, hold it in her hands on a regular basis envisioning it filling with her class fee, keep it in a special place in her home. This would ground her intention into the physical. It would no longer simply be an energetic desire.

She would call from time to time and report her progress. The extra money was coming from unexpected places, but other emergencies kept coming up with the children that required she remove and use some of it. I kept assuring her that it would be there at the perfect time for her to receive Reiki training.

It took almost one year before the phone rang and she excitedly exclaimed, "I did it, I've got $150 and I can now register for the next class!"

Two months after her Reiki initiations I answered the phone and would never have known it was the same person, she sounded so much healthier and full of life. Her confidence level was high. In a new loving, gentler voice she said, "I had to call you…I have $500 for my Second Degree training and am doing lots of self-treatment, in addition to treating clients and receiving Reiki from other practitioners. Now with the three months minimum period between classes I will practice more and dream of the day of my next level of training."

Then there was the 27-year-old student who brought me her completed application to become a Reiki Master Candidate. While responding to the question regarding how she wished to pay the $10,000 fee for her training, she started her answer: "I will—Just for today, do not worry."

When students commit to living the life of a Reiki Master, it is recommended that they quit their current employment so they have the time for Reiki and can truly surrender to the energy of Reiki supporting them in every way. From experience, I believe those that don't do this miss out on tremendously powerful lessons and benefits derived from the excitement of the wisdom gained.

One of Mrs. Takata's masters recently told me, "Reiki Masters can do as much Reiki as they want. Depends on how much you want your own life. I can continue to go all around the world with Reiki but I now choose to sit home with my grandchildren."

Unlimited Abundance

Reiki may not be for everyone because there are no guarantees of how it will work for any given individual, and it often becomes an entirely new way to look at life. The irony is that our life patterns move in cycles and what we think is a new way of life may actually be a way that was practiced before in the past.

For me, when I found a way to have unlimited abundance in all aspects of my life, just by getting my mind out of the way and keeping my Reiki Hands on my body, year after year I could find no reason to want it any other way.

There is nothing kept from you that you have not kept from yourself.

Our quiet inner voice is more intelligent than our thinking mind. Trust and Surrender are the first lessons Reiki teaches us as we continue the steps on our journey.

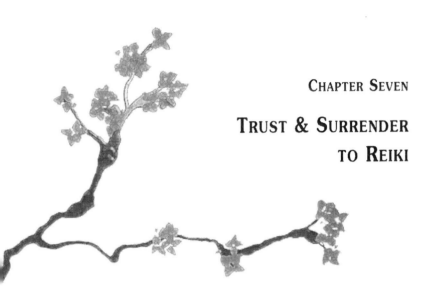

CHAPTER SEVEN

TRUST & SURRENDER TO REIKI

Ahhh yes—the old Trust and Surrender process. How did we get so far away from it?

Ever notice how many different understandings there are of a simple basic truth of life?

When did we start thinking we need to control everyone and everything that shares our space?

Why do so many individuals truly believe they are the only ones who know the right way?

We plow through project after project, person after person, wondering why everyone doesn't think the same way we do.

"No work no gain" has been a common saying in our society. How quickly we forget the principle that once we envision or state our intentions, then release our hold on them, more often than not, what we intend comes to fruition.

Reiki Makes Us Alive On A New Level

Trust and Surrender are the first lessons Reiki teaches us. In the beginning, as I heard the words Reiki Natural Healing, I connected with the vibration. My inner knowing was to trust it as something for further investigation.

When a friend suggested making an appointment for a treatment, I did. I surrendered to my gut feeling that it was going to be a good thing for me. No dramatic healing seemed to take place during the first treatment, but for some inexplicable reason I found myself quickly making appointments for more sessions. Incredibly, I just knew and trusted it was the next step to take.

Because Reiki works at such profound healing levels, this is often the case for people after connecting with its energy. At first the healing was subtle. Then I noticed my intuition coming alive on a new level, and my physical body seemed to be waking up.

There was a new heightened awareness of all my senses; colors appeared more vibrant; I began hearing new and different tones; I perceived aromas I hadn't noticed before; I started discovering a more refined taste in food and drink; various textures of things around me took on new meaning.

I was feeling a connection to the source of all things in a totally new way.

For many people, receiving Reiki is quite an innovative experience and the results of treatment may not be what they expected. For instance, a typical situation that requires healing is when you experience pain; you would probably pop a pill or go to a medical doctor, then, with medication, the pain may subside. This instant pain relief may not happen after a Reiki session because Reiki's main focus is to heal the cause, not "band-aid" the discomfort.

Reiki Natural Healing teaches how vitally important it is

to listen respectfully to messages the body is communicating. Our body is trying to tell us lifestyle changes need to be made if we truly want to heal. These valuable messages may come in the form of deep physical, emotional or spiritual healing.

Our return to the wholeness process can take a completely different route while the causes of our discomforts are being healed. As we have more of these Reiki healing occurrences, we learn to trust and surrender to the all-knowing, inexhaustible source of the energy moving through us, Reiki!

A Second Degree student once said in class: "I can't do everything. So I just do one thing! Trust in Reiki—the source that sustains me."

No Expectations — No Disappointments!

Reiki treatments repeatedly provide clients relief and healing with energy medicine. Once in awhile, however, during or after treatment (more often with chronic conditions) the pain may amplify before letting go, resulting in a deeper healing release.

The benefits of treatment in chronic conditions may not be immediately obvious, so it can be difficult for the client to understand and accept the process initially. This is when it is important to realize how long it took to create the situation. Layers of physical, emotional mental and spiritual healing may need to take place to achieve lasting results. Trust and surrender to Reiki's divine process are needed during these times.

The norm during Reiki treatment is relaxation, and yet when emotional healing is taking place, the mind may become very active while outmoded and no longer needed thought forms are being purged and the physical and emotional bodies are readjusting themselves. To receive full enjoyment and benefits from Reiki treatments, it is best not to have expectations.

This is the case in all we experience throughout life. No expectations—no disappointments! Holding on to a desire to control things in life can get in the way of and prevent wonderful healing surprises from happening.

Reiki Training Offers Healing Like No Other

After graduating from understanding the importance of trust and surrender during Reiki treatment, the next level of your healing may be working with the process through Reiki training.

Years ago, while driving to my First Degree Reiki class, many thoughts were surfacing for healing. As hard as it is to believe now, at that time my family and friends didn't do a lot of touching. Nor did they as I was growing up. Hugs were certainly not as common place with me as they are today. So the mere thought of placing my hands on someone I didn't know in the training was an unpleasant feeling I had to surrender to.

Comforted by my determination to receive the tool of self-treatment, I continued on. The desire to provide treatments for other people or to take Second Degree training was not of the least interest to me then. Reiki at times seems to dangle a golden carrot in front of us, guiding us in the next direction needed for our overall health and well being. Typically, I've found it is best not to know what the next step is until the one at hand is addressed. It seems to open the door somehow to what lies ahead.

My first day of class was unbelievable. As I gently placed my hands on the head of the partner I was working with, her headache was eliminated! I couldn't help but think of Jesus doing this and saying, "Go forth and do as I do." My hands felt they were radiating out love every moment—and they were.

After searching for a long time for the unknown something that was missing in my life, I had finally found it! There was a feeling of completeness as I felt a reconnection to the source of all life. With that connection came the most profound expression of love. I was in love with everyone and everything with no need to know why! I was surprised at that moment to realize how little of my life had been blessed with such meaningful moments.

Later in class, as I was receiving a full Reiki treatment, it became clear why I had cried through one of my first Reiki sessions. I could never remember receiving that level of love before. Yes, this was without a doubt what I had always been searching for without even knowing it. Because I wasn't probing to understand with my logical mind, I trusted and surrendered to the guidance of my heart—and this allowed me to receive one of the greatest gifts of my life.

As soon as time would allow, I took Second Degree training and knew then I would one day become a Reiki Master. Deep inside I wanted more people to know about and receive the benefits of this simple, powerful, healing modality. How could Reiki Natural Healing not bring more peace, love and energetic balance to our planet and her people?

The concept of sending healing energy to someone located in a different place quickly stirred up more lessons of surrender regarding trust. Could this connection possibly be made? Am I just making this up—is it really happening? How can the healing energy be sent to another and to someone I didn't even know?

When students in the class sent Reiki healing to the same person and shared our reports of the things experienced, it was astounding to discover that where I had noted blocked energy was actually a problem area. How was this possible? Repeated validations allowed me to surrender and trust that I didn't have to understand it intelligibly for it to be possible.

Self-Treatment Is The Foundation Of The Practice

It wasn't easy to get in the habit of giving myself time in the morning and evening for self-treatment. At first I would simply forget about it and then later try to catch up. As the habit started to feel pretty good, then better and better, I realized I needed less sleep, my schedule was flowing effortlessly throughout the day, and synchronicities were becoming commonplace. I felt respect for myself on a new level, didn't get sick anymore and felt more alive than I could ever remember feeling before.

I realized by then that I wouldn't dream of not doing self-treatment. When you know that Reiki provides huge benefits and feels so wonderful, why would you not treat yourself to the divine gift by simply placing your hands on yourself and allowing the healing energy to flow? Soon I found my hand going into a Reiki position automatically as I was driving, on the telephone or computer, in a meeting or movie, or on an airplane. Whenever a hand was free, I allowed it to give me a Reiki energy boost by simply placing my hand on my body.

Saying the Reiki Precepts as needed throughout the day and during self-treatment added an entirely new dimension to the process. The Precepts are a complete healing story within themselves. When I first heard them in class they seemed like simple words, and then I wanted to change and update them by coming from a more positive perspective. Soon their power and my respect for the way they were originally presented started to become obvious. To this day, I am continually humbled by the understanding and emotional healing they are able to bestow upon us.

Giving Reiki Treatments

When the time came, it was such an honor to feel that I

was prepared to provide Reiki treatments for other people in a professional manner.

My Master had told me, "When you are ready it will happen naturally." She added, "I would like you to experience having paid clients before taking your Second Degree training."

What a challenge that was! I was making plenty of money in the corporate world and didn't feel a need for the funds. I couldn't understand why she felt this was important, especially when the clients coming for treatment seemed to be struggling financially. After trusting and surrendering to the practice it didn't take long to appreciate what an important part of their healing it was for them to make an effort, a true commitment to their healing process.

It was becoming clear to me that no one can heal another; they need to accept their own healing responsibility. Only then can lasting healing take place. It also taught me to value my time and efforts and respect Reiki Natural Healing on an even deeper level.

An ongoing lesson was shared with me when one of my first clients so gently put it in plain words, "The only thing that is free is nothing, a no-thing. A 'no-thing' is something that doesn't exist. If it is something then it has a value. A something in the higher realms is never given for free because that would demote it to the level of a no-thing thereby destroying its right to exist in its present form. It would return to raw energy."

She further explained, "Whenever we encounter a product or service that claims it is free, we intuitively understand that somewhere someone is still paying the bill."

I did a lot of contemplating on these valuable words.

I continue to have incredible experiences with Reiki working in many powerfully diverse ways and often times not in the manner the client or I are expecting. And yet it is an ongoing process that is so brilliantly clear; the energy knows what the next perfect step is for that individual's healing process. To this day I remain fascinated and amazed at the unlimited possibilities of Reiki energy medicine.

Reiki Mastery

First Degree training introduced me to a new world full of exciting possibilities. Second Degree took a lot of trust to accept the certainty about distant healings working so exceedingly well. There was no comparison though to the surrender needed while learning to understand Reiki during master training, or how Reiki initiations could possibly work each and every time.

How was it that I could perform a simple ceremony and reawaken healing energy within someone's hands? How could the initiations automatically create a reliable and precise flow of healing energy with no transference of personal energy? What an exceptionally humbling honor to be merely a funnel for this loving life force energy coming through me.

Now as a full-time Reiki Master for many years, I am aware of my ever expanding opening to trust and surrender as I move forward in my understanding of healing, spiritual growth and personal development on deeper and deeper levels.

I can easily notice when and what issues are up for me in my personal never ending healing process, while recognizing that clients and students divinely guided to come to me are on some level mirror imagines of the next layer of what is up for me to heal. Reiki works with our overall healing process and teaches us how to serve our students and clients in a more pure and whole way.

Reiki's divine process allows me to know clearly how to understand my clients and student, because I am living their healing experiences with them. After treatments and trainings, to recognize the gift you have shared with them—well, there just couldn't be anything more gratifying. What a reward it is to witness students connecting with Reiki for the first time and to know that when they leave the class they will have a powerful tool to assist them and others to live healthier, happier lives.

Reiki Brings Us What We Are Ready To Handle

Sometimes life presents huge new challenges as we learn to honor the divine process of this world and her people. Hurricane Iniki hit our island of Kauai at 175 miles per hour on Aloha Friday, September 11, 1992 at 1:28 p.m. Past lessons I had learned in trust and surrender were zilch to what was experienced during this natural island wide disaster. It was mind-boggling at the time and yet today I am so grateful for the deep healing perspective it provided.

On Thursday, the day before Iniki's visit, it became clear that we would be hit hard by the hurricane. My phone rang and it was an invitation from some island healers to join them in their energy work to direct the hurricane winds in another direction. I responded that I didn't know if I could do that but I would send Reiki to Iniki and get back with them. It was an awesome experience because the meaning of the word Iniki is "piercing sword." And yet during my distant Reiki connection I was receiving a tremendously loving influence. I asked the energy if it would not come to Kauai, and it responded that it was sorry but it was a necessary part of a natural cleansing action. It told me no one would be hurt unless they hurt themselves. Out of approximately 50,000 people, and who knows how many more tourists, only three people lost their lives and few injuries were reported. My understanding was that the few deaths were not as a direct result of the hurricane.

The connections that were made among our island people were heartwarming and needed. Neighbors that had never met were helping each other in any way they could. People who had extra food, water, blankets or whatever placed items in front of their homes for those that needed them. Markets were without electricity to keep their freezers running, generously offered the frozen items to their island family.

The morning of the hurricane a client from Egypt called and asked if he could keep his 10 a.m. Reiki treatment appointment. Trusting that things were happening in Divine Order, I agreed to see him, three hours before the disaster was to occur. There was unbelievably remarkable energy present and it empowered me to a new level of mastership. As if it were yesterday, I remember looking out my large picture window at beautiful flowers and birds and sensing the stillness that only happens before a storm while I moved my hands from position to position providing a healing treatment for the two of us. At 11:30 a.m. the client was on his way to secure himself while there was still time.

My home was a two-story house with many large windows. Most everyone was encouraging me to go to the local shelter. I had mixed emotions about it so sat down and sent Reiki to the situation. It was clear that I was to stay put and surrender to the process. The energy guided me to collect food and lots of water, place a lounge pad on the floor of my large walk-in closet upstairs and Reiki myself to sleep, which somehow I managed to do. Upon awaking I could hear the storm blowing through the house. Peeking out the closet door, I saw my CD's flying by. The only thing to do was to give myself more self Reiki treatment and wait for things to calm down.

It was beyond belief to see the damage. The winds had entered one upstairs bedroom window. A large portion of that window was stuck half in and half out of the partial wall between the bedroom and living room below. Talk about piercing sword!

The winds of change had moved down into the living room, took a right turn and went to the corner where Reiki materials and books were on display, picked up most everything, then left out that corner of the house and distributed Reiki information all over the island. But in the end, there was little damage to the house while some homes around me were completely destroyed.

Reiki students and friends arrived and assisted to put things back in order before taking the Reiki tables and finding our way through the debris to the Red Cross relief site to provide much needed Reiki treatments for our grateful island community. We were given a room next to the Red Cross medical area and worked hand in hand for days with their staff. I learned so much valuable information about the miracles of Reiki Natural Healing in disaster situations. Often we had one person after another on the Reiki table from 9 a.m. to 9 p.m. and yet at the end of the day we felt energized from receiving the treatments coming through us. Red Cross personnel took blood pressure readings then sent people for Reiki. The readings were always lower after their treatment.

Stress was off the scale for children who had been ignored while the adults couldn't keep up with or handle what had happened. To further complicate matters, a major hurricane, Andrew, hit Florida the month before, and some insurance companies had filed bankruptcy, leaving many of our residents unknowingly with no insurance.

We went from table to table giving mini treatments to personnel that were exhausted from assisting people to complete the mounds of required paperwork. There was no end to the situations where Reiki energy healing was needed and appreciated fully. Requests for Reiki continued to grow as our local radio station invited citizens to come and take advantage of our volunteer efforts. With no electricity or telephone service for days, the battery powered radios were our only source of information.

One day as things seemed to be settling on the island, I felt an urge to go to the local radio station that had been on the air 24/7 trying to help people survive this wearisome situation. Setting up my Reiki table in the recording studio, I started treating the staff. Boy, did they need and appreciate it!

I had surrendered to and trusted what had occurred since Iniki first paid us her visit. It was time for the disaster sites to shut down and our practitioners to get back to regular clients. The Red Cross was providing vouchers for medical treatment when several requests came through for Reiki Natural Healing. The nurse in charge explained that it was not an approved health service. So many people complained and wrote letters to receive treatment that it was finally approved for us to provide treatments and training and be reimbursed by the disaster funds. A complete treatment report was prepared for each client I treated and/or initiated into Reiki. Included with the reports were pages of positive documentation from those that had received Reiki Natural Healing. This information packet was submitted to the American Red Cross with the suggestion that Reiki be included as part of the disaster teams going into these crisis situations.

A Reiki Vacation

After the winds of change quit blowing it was clearly time for a much-needed rest. The energy was guiding me to visit the Hawaiian island of Molokai. This small relaxing, laidback island is considered the family island of the Hawaiian chain. Arriving at their tiny airport was rewarding, and to think I had a week to do nothing but enjoy this lush tropical paradise.

Distracted by meeting warm, loving, interesting people on the tiny airplane and in the airport, it wasn't until we were on a small bus several miles down the road that I realized I had left my suitcase back at the airport. The bus driver explained that his was the only bus taking people to the hotels and he would take me back, but not until he completed his rounds. This took awhile so we were becoming the best of friends in the process. With everyone delivered to their hotel we headed back to the airport when he asked if I would like to stop for a coconut. After previously sending Reiki to my bag I trusted that it was okay and surrendered to the situation.

As we sat under a large Banyan tree sipping from our coconuts, the driver explained his pain and health problems. Before long I was administering a mini Reiki treatment as he is sitting on a log in the shade under the tree.

It was almost dark when we arrived back at the little airport, which was now closed. There on the outside conveyer belt, all by itself, where anyone could have picked it up, was my suitcase waiting for me.

As the bus driver and I drove back to my hotel we passed a park area where he noticed some friends playing music, singing and just getting ready to have dinner. By this time we were both hungry so he stopped to "talk story" knowing we would be invited to enjoy their grinds (Hawaiian slang for food). Soon he was explaining to everyone how Reiki took his pain away and revitalized him after his tiring day. More lessons in trust and surrender as Reiki seeds were being planted on the island of Molokai!

The next day I was on a mule ride on the far north side of the island, trusting and surrendering to the bumpy ride while going down a steep hillside to a place called Kalaupapa. In 1865 eight thousand Hawaiians afflicted with leprosy (later named Hansen's Disease) lived and died there. Needless to say, the energetic influence on the area was intense. I felt directed to use Reiki in many locations to assist with clearing the energy and the land.

In 2001 while reading the August/September issue of Reiki Magazine I found myself smiling as I read an article by Reiki Master Jean Ferris. It told of an adventure she had with her twelve students in 1993, being guided to Kalaupapa to heal the living and the dead, the land and the spirits. I could relate. When Reiki Masters learn to truly trust and surrender to Reiki's guidance, it is clear that it isn't about giving up, it is about letting go. As we do so, life is never boring.

**Forget your past track record.
Each moment is a new beginning.**

*The greater the change; the greater is the growth
and rewards. This collection of tales is just a hint
of what Reiki can bring about in life.*

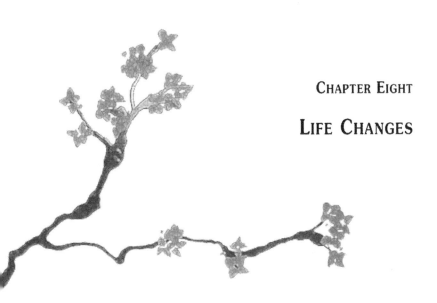

After Reiki training life changes begin happening. For some the changes may be slight, for me they have been like sticks of dynamite, one big charge after another blowing me out of my old ways and into new exciting adventures.

Reiki's curative energy often brings addictions to the surface for healing. Some we may have been unaware of, while others are obvious, such as cigarette smoking, alcohol and drug use, caffeine and junk food consumption, and there could be other things like addictive lifestyles we may have been completely oblivious to! Being overly lethargic or being a workaholic both are acute addictive lifestyles.

When the body is kept full of healing life force energy, unnatural ways and inappropriate substances noticeably don't taste as good, nor do they produce the same results and therefore are not nearly as appealing. The more one receives

Reiki's healing energy the more a natural and lasting high starts to take place, one that is similar to, but more than, seeing a rainbow or a beautiful sunset in nature.

Alcohol To Herb Tea

Reiki found me at a fascinating time. Life was good. I was living in an elegant home on the Gold course at Doral Country Club in Miami, Florida. Health problems were not an issue. I was active, loved playing golf and tennis and took pleasure in water skiing. My husband and I had a boat docked in Key Largo which we enjoyed as time permitted.

It wasn't until after Reiki training that I started to realize how much alcohol I was consuming. There were drinks at parties, at lunch with a customer or vender, after work drinks with friends to relax from a tiring day, wine with dinner, and occasionally a nightcap before going to sleep. It was shortly after I had started receiving Reiki treatments that someone mentioned to me, "If you put alcohol in your system every day you are an alcoholic." That thought hadn't even crossed my mind. That is the way Reiki works; at the perfect time in my healing process those were the exact words I needed to hear to clearly jolt my awareness and start focusing on discontinuing an unhealthy drinking habit I wasn't even aware I had.

Reiki energy shows us what to do away with, while guiding us to what is needed for our overall health. Plus, the more we work with the healing energy, the quicker it will assist us to remedy situations, often even before we know they are a problem. This happens on both conscious and unconscious levels, making Reiki Natural Healing an incredibly simple, yet powerful health maintenance tool.

Florida To Hawaii

New changes in our lives can be a bit scary, if we allow them to be. As we move from the warm fuzzy life we know so well into unfamiliar territory the ride can be a bit bumpy. Some of the more problematical changes arise when we discontinue long-standing patterns that are not for the highest good of our overall health. Usually those that shared them with us no longer appear interesting or fun to be around.

When friends become unappealing it can easily create a desire to relocate where the energy is more conducive to supporting our new life style. The in-between stage usually is the most difficult. The mind kicks in and creates logical excuses why we need to stay where we are established, while the heart begs us to leave and grow in new, more fertile soil. For awhile we may teeter-totter all alone in this life-changing void between old and new friends. If we don't understand or appreciate what is happening, it can be a really painful place to hang out. Comfort eventually returns on a new level after we surrender to the innovative healthier lifestyle being presented and allow the energy to truly guide and support the new process.

Personally, after Reiki training I was feeling so delightful about my new life changes I wanted my husband, two married daughters, sister, their families, and some of my friends to experience these amazing healing benefits too. It was shocking indeed to learn they had no interest. Of course, being a type "A" corporate personality at the time, one that knew only too well how to sell, I was a bit pushy in my excitement of discovering the treasures of Reiki. For some inexplicable reason, the more I tried to convince them to experience this newly found divine gift, the less interest they showed.

Life with my husband and friends changed so drastically that I had to remove myself from the environment that was no longer supportive to my healthier lifestyle. We were living totally different lives and now had little, if any, of the same interests to share. Albert Einstein, one of the most brilliant scientists in modern history, is known to have said, "No problem can be solved from the same level of consciousness that created it." It was clear to me that I had no desire to go back to my old level of consciousness.

After being a married woman since the age of sixteen and mother of two daughters before the age of twenty, I was truly stepping into the unknown. New life changes involved leaving my traditional family structure for the first time and corporate security as well. On top of all this, now I felt compelled to move to one of the most expensive places in the world to live the life of a Reiki Master.

As the airplane was landing in Honolulu I realized I was about as far away from Florida and family and friends as I could travel and still remain in the United States. It was not an easy time experiencing all the emotional highs and lows. And yet, there was a continual presence of complete validation, peace and underlying calm that comforted my soul.

When major life changes happen and we are able to keep our limited minds free of worry, there appears to be this all-knowing protective guidance directing us unerringly right back into the natural flow of life.

Even with lots of Reiki support, flying from Florida to Honolulu was physically and mentally exhausting. As I exited the airplane, warm gentle trade winds began caressing my hair. I took a deep breath inhaling the fresh ocean scent combined with the sweet fragrance of tropical flowers. I now had a new knowledge deep inside of me that these life changes were truly in Divine Order. How was it possible to suddenly feel at home when I had left behind my home, family and friends?

Incredible first time experiences centered on living independently in the world were coming to me. I realized I had never encountered little things that many people take for granted. For thirty of my forty-six years of life my husband had read the road maps, driven the car, made restaurant and hotel reservations and even filled the car with gasoline.

Fun, scary and exciting new lessons were quickly arising. Tears of joy filled my eyes as I watched happy people playing music and singing while welcoming me with open arms. Leis made of the most interesting flowers, shells, and yarns were placed around my neck.

One Sunday I was starting to feel a little lonely and wondered into an old Hawaiian church. A beautiful Hawaiian lady sitting next to me caught my attention. She was radiating out this new love energy, the very one that I was now determined to incorporate into each and every aspect of my life. What did she know that I wanted to know? I became more curious when she seemed to sense my anxiety and twinge of loneliness. A powerful, loving sensation came over me as she gently placed her hand on mine. She will never know how needed that simple gesture of aloha was at that exact moment in time. Recalling it continues to this day to open my heart and bring back a loving, comforting, sensation. At times I wonder if she had Reiki hands.

Each day in this new island heaven was bringing more joy and lightheartedness to my being. Hiking the outrageously beautiful trails in Hawaii was connecting me with the energies of nature like never before. Lava rocks, trees, plants, water and nature spirits were actually communicating with me in new and intriguing ways as we danced and played together.

My body sought to breathe, stretch, run, jump, swim; I couldn't seem to do it all fast enough. These life changes, supported by lots of Reiki were truly showing me how to fully experience the healing energy of a Hawaiian paradise. People were extremely friendly and helpful, not like acquaintances I had left behind so stressed, serious and worried about work and monetary things. Some days I would take pleasure in the new found joy of simply sitting in nature for hours alone or "talking story" with recently discovered friends.

The rental car took me all over the different islands, in

towns, housing areas, and sugar cane fields, up mountains and along the coastlines. There was so much to see and I wanted to experience it all. I was free; I was going to be living in Hawaii!

Kauai Calls

After making my way around and through each of the other five Hawaiian Islands, I found myself in a large Kauai home. When I initially spoke to the owner over the phone it sounded like a special deal so I rented it sight unseen. It was not as pleasant upon arrival as my mind had envisioned. The house required much cleaning and I was as yet unaware of the numerous little creatures that share your living space in the tropics. However, it was the perfect setting for my upcoming lessons and life changes to unfold.

I remember times of feeling alone, so far from family and friends, and yet there was a real unexplainable sense of completeness present. Reiki had become a friend like no other. It was a companion that was always there to provide calmness, clarity and guidance. With Reiki self-treatment along with the comfort of the Reiki Precepts, the old emotions of fear, worry and anger were melting away like magic, and I was soon reconnected to the joy of my new adventure.

One of my first lessons was about the real meaning of the word alone (all one). As the days passed I felt less alone than I had in the presence of family and friends on the mainland. How could this be possible? I discovered that even though we are alone doesn't mean we have to be lonely. We are in reality one with all of life. We came from and will return to the same place. As we grow and connect more with this oneness, there is a new wholeness that overcomes us. We actually find a new awareness of those things that before were unidentifiable—those things we thought were missing in our lives.

Being alone became less and less of an issue as old feelings of insecurity were falling away. When this happened, it allowed me to radiate out the new energy I wanted to attract into my life. Friends now were ones I could actually communicate with at a new, more loving level of consciousness.

As we learn to follow the energy of life, synchronistic occurrences become commonplace and life continues to get easier and easier to understand and enjoy. As we become healthier in body, mind and spirit, there is an incredible feeling of wholeness in our lives, no matter where we are or whom we are with.

Hospital Experience

My mother became ill during my high school years. At the age of fourteen I had visited her in the hospital during several weeks, watching her grow weaker and weaker, until she passed away. These visits left lasting memories of the unpleasant hospital atmosphere and caused me to spend my life avoiding hospitals as much as possible. It was becoming clear that it was time to heal these old outdated feelings and thought forms as Reiki clients were calling me into the hospital on a never ending basis. Soon, I had established a Reiki program at our local island hospital.

Once more, on a new level, Reiki Natural Healing was showing me the miraculous level of healing possible by simply filling one's body with life force energy. Through treatments, Reiki helped to amplify and support the staff and the patient's innate healing abilities. My students and I shared Reiki with several patients that were on high dosages of morphine and still in pain, unable to relax or sleep. After a calming Reiki treatment they were more often than not peacefully sleeping like a baby. We also provided Reiki before and after surgeries. It was gratifying to continually receive positive feedback about how smoothly the procedures went as well as amazing stories about the unusually rapid recovery time.

Frequently, people who have been sick for a while find relief in not having to deal with previous responsibilities at home and at work. Some start receiving love and attention they were missing in the past. Getting over illness can bring back some old and unwanted ways. Reiki healing creates life changes and brings to the surface for healing subconscious thought forms that are blocking physical healing. An awareness of this process may occur in many different ways; by a casual statement someone makes that suddenly triggers an emotional release, an article you read in the newspaper, radio broadcasts, other media, or even in the dream state.

A hospital Reiki program may extend an invitation for Reiki treatments, or there may be nights when your dreams clearly show what health changes are needed. Our Reiki hospital program on Kauai was established to include weekly visits to the Adult Day Care and Long Term Care areas. This proved to be a special way for practitioners to live our third Reiki Precept, "Honor your parents, teachers, and elders."

Unlimited Travel

Life changes around international travel began early in my Reiki Master years. We jokingly tell our Reiki Master candidates that one of the first things they may want to do is procure a passport. Later it becomes clear it was no joking matter. Taking into account expenses involved when traveling internationally with my husband, for one or two week vacations here and there, traveling as a Reiki Master was completely different.

In 1991 when I became a member of The Reiki Alliance I was puzzled about how masters could afford to travel to such exotic places for yearly conferences. After all, many had given up high paying job positions as I had to live the life of Reiki. And yet, when I signed the membership agreement, the requirement was to attend Regional Gatherings and the International Conference as often as possible. The time had come to work with this travel energy. I had no clue what was ahead of me in the upcoming months.

From Canada To Australia

It all started when I wanted to meet the lineage bearer of Reiki, Phyllis Furumoto. I received an invitation to attend a retreat at her property in Canada. While excitedly approaching the travel details via my old habits—checking flight costs and looking at where funds may be coming from—the word Australia continued to be in my face.

Being a new Reiki Master and not understanding the signs, I was in a state of bewilderment. Why, when I'm making plans to go to Canada, is Australia presenting itself when I turn on TV, pick up a magazine or even during conversations? I did mention a few years back that a trip "down under" would be terrific, but why now? Finally the energy of Australia became so intense I could no longer ignore it.

One day I sent Reiki to the situation and then opened a map of the area and said out loud, "Okay, if you want me to go, where in Australia am I to go?" The area of Perth located in Western Australia immediately jumped out at me. My heart's desire was to visit the action packed eastside— the Gold Coast. The energy wouldn't budge. There was no doubt about it; this was where I was going for who knows what reason.

Well, all sorts of interesting tales can be told about how I acquired the airplane ticket. Not until it was in my hand did I find out our Reiki lineage bearer would be in Perth for a conference during the time I would be there. This is only the very beginning and a tiny part of the story.

The next energy push was to give up Kauai. What? I had finally found the perfect spot in the world to live and the message was to sell my worldly possessions (a 20-foot container of stuff brought with me all the way from Florida). Not only that, this included my yellow mustang convertible which I brought with me and dearly loved. After lots of Reiki on everything involved, I surrendered part way by placing some personal goodies I couldn't bear to part with in storage. Then I had a huge garage sale that made many people on the island exceedingly happy.

Now picture this! I'm in my car with its new owner on the way to the airport and we stop at the post office for the last bit of mail I may see for some time. Hurriedly I placed it in my carry-on case. After clearing a few tears and saying good-bye to Kauai as the plane is flying off in the distance, I started to relax and take a look at the mail. Hmm, what is this? A manuscript titled Mutant Message by Marlo Morgan, a fellow UB minister. This is interesting; it appears to be about Australia.

Well, after reading the Mutant Message manuscript I didn't know whether to take the next plane to somewhere else or what! And sure enough, it wasn't long into my visit to Australia that I was out in the bush with the Aborigines. The synchronicities of events to get me there were all so enchanting.

At the time I purchased the ticket for this trip, the travel agent explained there was a free stop from Kauai to Western Australia and asked if I would like to visit any other destination. Thinking for only a moment, I inquired about New Zealand. A deep longing lingered inside me to visit the "land of the long white cloud." Next my thoughts went to Fiji and it wasn't long after that I found myself holding a ticket to all three places. And to think the energy that started all of this was to go to Canada and meet Phyllis Furumoto. Attempting to use your logical mind in these types of fascinating Reiki experiences simply won't work.

Fiji Islands

First stop was the islands of Fiji. It was so strange, because of the time difference I arrived there the day before I left

Hawaii. It felt as if I was living the same day twice. Talk about the "no such thing as time" concept of the ancients. A dear friend on Kauai made arrangements for me to stay with her brother's family in Lautoka. Not knowing anyone or anything about the area, I was most grateful to see him at the airport at 5 a.m. to greet my plane.

On the way to his home it was amazing to witness so many local people at such an early hour exercising by walking together. It didn't take long for it to become clear I needed this stop in Fiji. Things had happened so rapidly I had no awareness of how much physical and emotional stress I had undergone preparing to leave my beloved Kauai. At the recommendation of my host, I took a boat tour to a small nearby island. Our arrival was greeted by joyful singing of the Fijians. What a nurturing, peaceful place to gently unwind from my emotional and physical ordeal.

The next day I met a young cab driver from India who became a longtime friend. After awhile I just had to ask him where Reiki Natural Healing was most needed in the community. He drove me to The Old Peoples Home. I couldn't help notice its pleasant, peaceful appearance as we drove onto the property. The residents were tending small vegetable and flower gardens, and there were lots of large shade trees with chairs underneath filled with chatting people. The healthy ambiance continued inside the humble structures where brightly colored tropical print curtains were blowing gently in the open windows.

Quickly I thought of some of the elderly homes I had visited in the past, with locks on the closed-in structures, the smell of urine ever present throughout the residence, and some of the people looking like zombies from being overly drugged. What an improved contrast in healing environments this was! These people appeared healthy because they were keeping their connection to the all-sustaining life force energy of nature that is needed to maintain health. What a wonderful, cheerful place with so many lovely people.

Before I started sharing Reiki treatments, they even served me a meal (which I soon learned I was to eat with my hands) while I was being introduced to the staff and volunteers. Afterwards residents sat in a chair in front of their beds as I walked behind each one providing a few minutes of Reiki healing energy. Completing the women's home brought up feelings of immense gratitude for me before being escorted across the courtyard to the men's quarters. It was a humbling and gratifying experience for me as a Reiki Master that I will always remember. In fact, there was so much love exchanged with these people, I flew back to Fiji on my return trip for another visit of sharing Reiki with these newly found friends.

Living the life of Reiki is so special that every single experience in life becomes one of giving and receiving in balanced harmony. I really think this is the way we are meant to live life in order to maintain wellness in body, mind and spirit.

Another fond memory of Lautoka was sitting in the park watching school children going home from classes. All of a sudden several of them were sitting cross legged in front of my park bench. I guess they were attracted to the Reiki energy and my blond hair and my white skin did gave away the fact that I was a visitor. They looked up at me with those sparkling dark black eyes as I noted their very dark skin and simply asked, "Tell us what it is like to live in America."

New Zealand

Next stop on this life changing Reiki expedition was Auckland, New Zealand. As much as I love island life I was ready for some first class excitement. It had been many months since I was wined and dined in the Miami country club atmosphere.

At the airport phone calls to other Reiki Masters were uneventful. With eyes closed, I pointed my finger to a hotel on the map, called and made a reservation, then walked out of the airport to a bus that made the rounds to local hotels. Surprisingly, I found myself walking to the back of the bus, which I seldom do, and taking a seat in front of the large rear window. Looking down at the people boarding the bus, a man in a white suit and hat caught my attention. He appeared attractive, and for just a second the thought passed my mind that I wouldn't mind exploring Auckland with him as my tour guide.

Going back to reading the tour book, I grinned at my thinking and was completely startled when I heard someone ask if the seat next to me was taken. Sure enough it was the man I had just admired outside the window. We do need to be careful what we think. To make a long story shorter, he offered to show me the city, which was just what I needed and it was totally delightfully first class.

The following day found me in the home of a Maori Reiki Master, which lead to many more Reiki contacts and new friendships. A few months later, I even taught a Reiki class there that I enjoyed so much sharing with these magnificent people. It was intriguing to discover, during my various visits all around North Island, the similarities of the Hawaiian and Maori cultures. I was told that long ago they left the same place and went in different directions in their outrigger canoes.

Australia

Next I was off to Melbourne, Australia to teach a Reiki class. This was before cell phones and the organizer hadn't been able to catch up with me in my travels. The class didn't come together, and it was the coldest day they had seen in over one hundred years! I found a hotel with the largest jacuzzi bathtub available, and spent most of the day in a hot bubble bath to stay warm. Touring Melbourne and sharing Reiki there would simply have to happen at a later date.

Not knowing what fate had in store for me, the next day I changed my ticket to arrive in Perth earlier than expected. Because of the extra time this change provided before the Reiki conference, I made arrangements to visit with a Reiki Master in Kalgoorlie for a few days before we attended the conference together. Not long after I had unpacked my things in his guestroom, he introduced me to some of his friends who were planning to show me the area while he handled his work commitment. This is when, by a turn of unexpected events, I ended up at a Bush Station for a few days connecting with Aborigines.

It didn't take long to discover what those things hanging down from some of the hats you see Aussies wearing were all about. Western Australia's outback has the most annoying flies I've ever experienced. As you walk, the pieces of leather hanging down from the hat sways and shoos the flies away. Those flies crawl and stick on you like glue, in your eyes, ears and nose. They really were my teacher and tested me on our fifth Reiki Precept to "show gratitude to every living thing."

As I was returning to the Bush Station one day from a "walk about" I asked what was hanging in the tree by the campfire and was told it was dinner. Later to my dismay, I tried my first taste of kangaroo. Because I was so hungry, I gave it a lot of Reiki and asked to receive dispensation from my vegetarian ways. Days in the bush were like none other. What joyful, loving, learning, experiences they turned out to be. My connection with nature and natural healing were rapidly moving to new, more profound levels of attentiveness. What a gift!

Even now, it isn't easy for me to believe that I didn't make it back to the Reiki Master's home where I had left all my belongings. It was most embarrassing to call my most gracious host and ask him to please be so kind as to pack my personal effects, and bring them to the conference.

Flying into Perth late at night in a small plane with new friends from the bush, I suddenly realized I had no idea where the conference the next morning was being held. My registration papers were with my other items in a car somewhere on their way to the conference, I hoped!

My new friend Tracey whom I had met in the bush invited me to spend the night. She started making phone calls to locate the conference and finally did so. She also loaned me some clean clothes to wear, as my unexpected trip to the bush lasted much longer than anticipated and I had been wearing the same clothes throughout my stay. Not a good thing! Finally, the time had come and I was to meet Phyllis Furumoto our Grand Master and attend the conference! It was all very enjoyable and the beginning of another lifelong friendship.

Looking up from our conversation, I saw the Reiki Master I had deserted and who I barely knew entering the conference carrying all my baggage. Now this was a lot of stuff because, at this point, I was planning to live in Australia for as long as the energy felt right to stay. I'm sure to this day he doesn't know what to think of this person who mysteriously came to visit then disappeared after just a couple of hours.

It was truly exhilarating to meet so many gracious masters as they extended invitations to stay with them in various places around Western Australia. So I followed the Reiki guidance and visited my new Reiki Master friends. As Reiki would have it, I found myself teaching classes in Perth. It was the one place that popped out at me when I opened the map of Australia not so very long ago. Going south to Albany I reconnected with a Reiki Master couple, Gloria and Graham, whom I had previously met at a Reiki get-together in Honolulu. Then they had come to visit Kauai where we enjoyed presenting Reiki Introductions together. I was also a guest in the lovely home of a magnificent Reiki Master couple in Perth, Hazel and Rod and their family.

Heading North I met Meg, a Reiki Master in Geraldton. She decided to take me to visit the dolphins and share Reiki with her students in Monkey Mia. We have fond Reiki memories of our morning attempt to get out of town. There seemed to be radiator problems with Meg's car and her mechanic suggested we not drive it over the weekend and return with it first thing Monday morning.

Being two strong Reiki Masters, the limits of this blocked energy didn't set well with us, we decided to go anyway. After all, what more could we need than lots of water and our Reiki hands? If I hadn't been there I wouldn't have believed it. Using the first Precept, "Just for today, do not worry," so our worry thoughts didn't create our reality, we watched the car's temperature gauge move towards the hot side. Immediately sending Reiki energy while placing a healing symbol over the top of the car, slowly we watched the gauge move towards cool. This happened more than a few times on the trip, as we balanced out the energy, until arriving safely at our destination. What a place it was!

The custom had begun here several years earlier by one person feeding the dolphins. Then, more dolphins and more people came to the area and now it is quite a well-known destination for visiting dolphins in Western Australia.

There was luscious healing energy present while sharing Reiki treatments with Meg and her students. It must have been even more powerful for her to have the privilege of providing initiations in such an energetic location in nature. She mentioned that some initiations had even been performed on the beach near the dolphin doorway. This was the sacred spot she selected for me to ordain her as a minister of the Universal Brotherhood Movement, an inter-faith non-denominational ministry enjoyed by healers from around the world.

As we drove along the road, I couldn't help noticing the bars attached to the front of everyone's vehicles. When I

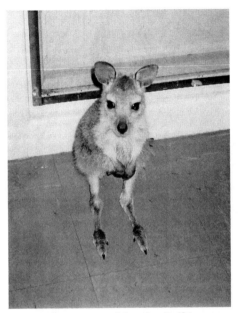

Kangaroo asking for Reiki

asked about them, Meg laughed and explained they were to protect the autos from the kangaroos crossing the roads at night. My first thought was, so what is protecting the animals from those who built the roads in their pathway? When a mother kangaroo is hit and killed, her pouch is so safe, the little one is normally alive inside and is taken into homes to be cared for until it is old enough to survive on its own.

My sadness grew when I entered the next home I was to visit. They had a "joey," a baby kangaroo living in their home just like a pet dog or cat. It was so clever—in the evening they would hold a bag similar to the old-fashioned clothespin bag in front of the joey and he would turn a little summersault in the air and land feet first inside, just as he had in his momma's pouch. The bag was then hung for the baby's restful sleep. I quickly discovered that baby kangaroo's love Reiki too.

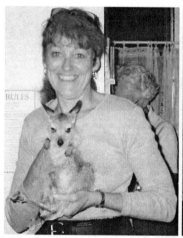 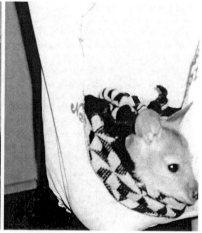

Kangaroo receiving Reiki   **Kangaroo resting after Reiki**

I purchased an Aussie bus pass and again headed off into the unknown to visit Reiki Masters in Exmouth, Port Hedland, and Broome, all the way up north to Darwin. As the bus pulled into Darwin I couldn't help exclaiming out loud "Plumerias!" The flowers have a different name there but how wonderful to experience them at the exact time I was missing Hawaii.

Before long I found myself at Uluru (Ayers Rock), a remarkable energy spot on the planet. It is a site to behold; the enormous rock appears to change colors several times as the sunlight hits it during the time of the setting sun. I've heard the colors change in the morning with the raising sun too, but not being a morning person I can't say for sure.

Another lesson in trust and surrender to the flow of the energy occurred as I was climbing the steep side of Ayers Rock. There seemed to be no breeze and yet my camera case, which was secure before the climb, came loose and blew side-ways off the trail. It looked as if it was asking me to follow. Each time I reached down to pick it up it would blow further away. Soon it had taken me to a beautiful place tucked away out of tourist sight. A little waterfall was hidden from the trail where ancient pictures adorned the rocks and the entire area gave off a blue glow. What a gift and lesson in our first Precept, "Just for today, do not worry."

Following a didgeridoo concert the next day, I was on another bus to Adelaide where I had a date with a special man. A 95 year old scientist and author with whom I had been corresponding told me of his days living in California and of his meeting Hawayo Takata, our third Reiki Grand Master and lineage bearer. He said he had not been ready for Reiki at that time, but now he wanted to receive First Degree training. What an adventure we experienced together. He had very little hearing left and couldn't see well, so during most of his private class I found myself screaming right in front of his face for him to see and hear. We had become pen pals and now the best of friends, walking down the street holding hands, on our way to lunch. In his favorite restaurant he proudly introduced me to his friends as his Reiki Master.

After three months of Reiki leading me all over the western half of Australia, it was clear that I had accomplished what needed to be done and I wasn't actually moving there. With renewed enthusiasm, I made arrangements to return to Kauai, by way of New Zealand and Fiji of course. Returning to those charming places and adding more friends to the new ones I had been blessed with are fabulous life-long memories.

And can you believe all of these life changes were allowed to happen because of following Reiki's guidance and not persisting to purchase the ticket to go to Canada, or refusing to give up Kauai? If anyone had predicted this journey was coming up in my life when I was working in the corporate world it would have been totally unbelievable. Could I have planned such a trip on my own without this energetic assistance? I don't think so!

Pizza Man In Oregon To Reiki Practitioner In Sedona

Significant life changes don't just happen to Reiki Masters. As an example, a client from Oregon walked into the studio in Kapaa for his first Reiki treatment. He connected well with the energy of Reiki and registered for training. When it was time to leave Kauai he wondered how he could take his Second Degree training from me. I told him if it was meant to be, Reiki would handle the details.

He was the owner of a Pizza restaurant in the town of Seaside near Portland and commented that he was not pleased with the clientele it was drawing. After returning home he called from his pizza place and I could hear loud Dixieland band music playing. My suggestion was to fill the restaurant with Reiki to assist with settling the energy, then start playing soothing Reiki music. He did and then began to draw the customers he truly enjoyed. It wasn't long afterwards that our Reiki Alliance conference was being held in Portland, at which time I went to Seaside and he received his Second Degree training.

The next word from him was notification that his business was for sale and he was going to massage school. Soon after that he was living in Sedona, Arizona happily experiencing his life changes providing massage and Reiki treatments.

Becky To Rebecca

In 1997 a young lady named Becky walked into a Reiki introduction I was having in Kapaa. She had broken up from an unpleasant relationship on Maui and came to Kauai with her daughter for healing. She wanted so much to take the training, but didn't feel she had the funds to do so. In the days to follow, she called and I would coach her on how to work with the energy of money. Soon the phone call came when I heard her excited voice exclaiming she had done it and would be in the class! Many changes occurred in her life with the support of Reiki. She moved back to Colorado and we stayed in contact.

In 1999 Becky's expected phone call came and she announced that she was ready for Second Degree training. Before long she had made arrangements to return to Kauai for the next scheduled class. As I recognized the energy shifts and positive life changes that had occurred for Becky just since our last phone conversation, I was overcome with excitement. Verifying her new self-empowerment, as I added her name to the class list she said, "Oh, by the way my name is now Rebecca."

It was further verified when, with her unmistakable new power following the Second Degree initiation, she noticed pictures of a student I had recently initiated a Reiki Master at beautiful Hanalei Bay on Kauai's plush north shore and said without hesitation, "One day I'll be back and would like to be initiated a Reiki Master at that location."

In 2002 there was another call from Rebecca. "I'm ready." She said, "Will you send me the application for Reiki Master Candidacy?" During her Master training she was organizing classes in Boulder and her ten-year-old daughter, Olivia, and boyfriend Paddy were initiated First Degree practitioners. Later Paddy asked her to marry him. She explained she would be going through a lot of changes during the training and after becoming a master. If he still felt he wanted to marry her after she was initiated she would love to do so. It was a beautiful year and a half of deeper bonding and training before Rebecca returned to Kauai for her Master initiation. It was in July on her thirty-sixth birthday, at the same place she had seen a few years earlier in the picture. In October she was married and is currently providing treatments and teaching classes primarily in Vermont and Colorado. www.ReikiBoulder.com

Painter To Reiki Practitioner

I have fond memories of another young client from Rio de Janeiro who came for his first Reiki treatment. Afterwards as he was getting off the Reiki table, he looked at me and remarked, "Wow, if I can get this high without using drugs, I want to learn Reiki." Here is another interesting case of how, when the student is ready, Reiki will find you in whatever form needed to get your attention.

This beautiful Brazilian man came to Kauai to assist with the island's recovery after the intense damage from Hurricane Iniki. He was working as a painter in one of the largest hotels on the island. Our local newspaper had recently printed a two-page story with pictures about our Reiki community. And lo and behold, the newspapers were used on the floor to protect it from the paint. It seemed no matter where he was painting, he would look down and our Reiki pictures were there, stirring his interest.

He noticed at lunchtime as he sat down to eat there was the Reiki article once again on the table right alongside him. After finally reading it, he called and said he felt he was destined to have a treatment, and after the session had no doubt that he wanted to take the class scheduled for the upcoming weekend. He registered before leaving, then called the next day in disappointment, saying in his excitement he had forgotten his girlfriend's birthday was on Saturday and she had things she wanted to do. I recommended he share with her the Reiki book he had purchased from me after his treatment. Soon he called back with renewed enthusiasm registering his girlfriend for the class too, and on the weekend we not only celebrated their introduction to Reiki Natural Healing, but a lovely birthday cake as well.

Waitress To Forest Ranger To Reiki Master

The Reiki Precepts are taught during the first day of class. While teaching in Colorado one year, a young lady returned the second day and explained to us that she had quit her waitress job that day because she realized she wasn't being fair to herself in how she was earning her living. She wasn't "Earning her Living Honestly."

She explained that financially she was okay until the first of the month when rent was due. Even after many years of teaching, I continue to be surprised at some occurrences in the classes. As calmly as possible I asked what she would like to be doing to earn her living. She was very moved by the flow of the healing energy and responded that she loved to dance and paint and would look for something in those areas even though her degree was in environmental studies.

After returning home to Kauai I received a phone call from Stefanie who exclaimed, "I am so happy, I now have a job doing what I've always wanted to do. I'm a forest ranger!" She continues to connect deeply with Reiki as each positive life change guides her along the healing pathway. Stefanie is no longer a forest ranger, we continued her training and now she is a successful full-time Reiki Master providing treatments and training in Denver, Colorado. www.ReikiDenver.com

Corporate World To Minister

Not only did my life changes include working with healing hands, they also included being ordained as an interfaith non-denominational minister, as well as a minister/director for the Universal Brotherhood Movement, Inc.

Several years ago in the state of Florida, Reiki practitioners were being told they needed to have a massage license or be a minister to legally practice Reiki. Since Reiki Natural Healing has nothing to do with massage, there was no interest in going through a year of massage training, and so we were without recourse.

Rick and Jeni Prigmore found other healing services were in a similar predicament. They went to an attorney and created a ministry. Universal Brotherhood Movement Inc. is an association composed of persons who have requested recognition of their independent ministries and have been officially ordained by U.B.M., Inc. Each minister conducts his or her ministry independently in the manner they deem fitting and proper and in accordance with local statutes.

I consider Reiki Natural Healing my ministry, as it is the best way I have found to help make this a healthier, happier world. UB also gives me the privilege to apply to the state for a license to perform weddings and other creative ceremonies, which I love to do out in nature, especially on the many beautiful beaches of Hawaii. It also provides a deeper connection with Reiki practitioners who use the services for their wedding and later for baptizing the baby, vow renewals, funerals or home and business blessings. What an awe-inspiring gift!

At times Reiki has become a valuable tool for assistance in creating personalized ceremonies. When requested, I use the distant healing method of connecting energetically with a couple to clarify what energy is best expressed for their wedding or celebration of life ceremony. It has also proven successful in connecting with an individual's energy to bring forth a christened name to be presented during a baptismal ceremony. More times than not in Hawaii, a Hawaiian name comes forth.

With UB and Reiki—there are no limits. I can assist those from any religious background, or those with no religious affiliation. The minister/director position provides the honor of ordaining others into this beautiful family of healers, which I often do while traveling. What a privilege it is to have introduced UB in Australia.

In fact several ordinations have been conducted at our Reiki Alliance conferences around the globe. Hawayo Takata was ordained a healing minister and she suggested it for some of her students. At the Portland Reiki Alliance conference mentioned earlier in this chapter, one of Takata's students honored her master's request to become a minister when I ordained her during the conference. Also during the event I had the privilege of ordaining Fokke, a Reiki Master who went home to Greece and later became a UB minister/director conducting ordinations there and other places. He now holds the distinction of introducing UB in Russia. UB now has ordained ministers in many countries around the world. The minister's card can be shown to those who may question our legal right to assist someone with their healing process. UB asks you to "Be true to your inner guidance" and encourages you to "Reach out and touch the earth and her inhabitants with love, compassion and responsibility." The UBM website address is: www.universalbrotherhood.org

As Reiki practitioners continually working with the healing energy, our life changes are ongoing. Life was never meant to be a hardship. Change is growth and the greater the change, often the greater the growth. The excitement escalates as you continue to recognize the only limits in life are self-created. What freedom this acknowledgment provides!

**Fear is the mind-talk that prevents
you from hearing your intuition.**

At this point in the journey we realize that limits are simply exciting opportunities. Reiki's healing energy seems to introduce itself to people at exactly the right time and in exactly the right way.

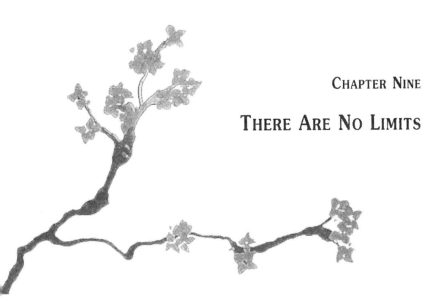

CHAPTER NINE

THERE ARE NO LIMITS

Sometimes when we are alone we send a call out into the universe, perhaps doubting if it was even heard. Later as the call is answered, we may have entirely forgotten about ever sending it. Experience has shown me over and over again that those drawn to Reiki simply have an inner knowing that on some level this is what they have been calling into their lives. Clients and students usually come to Reiki at a time when they are really ready to make positive changes in all areas of their life.

When You Are Ready to be a Reiki Student Reiki Will Find You

More often than not, when the divine timing is right, the word Reiki comes in unexpected ways. The mind doesn't always understand but the heart simply knows deep within

that it is something important to pay attention to. Perhaps
Reiki comes to us though a book, a dear friend or a dream. For
some it is a feeling of being drawn to Reiki without even knowing what it is. Reiki's healing energy seems to use no limits to
introduce itself to people.

Fond memories flood my mind and are accompanied by a
gentle chuckle when I recall a funny story that began on the
tennis courts of the old Coco Palms Hotel on Kauai. It was a
beautiful Hawaiian day and I was participating in a round-
robin-mixed-doubles tournament. Afterwards the gentleman
from the other side of the court inquired about my profession.
I said, "I'm a Reiki Master." He replied, "Oh really? I love (I
thought he said Reiki)."

His response prompted an invitation to join our get-
together that evening. Sitting around the Reiki tables about
to commence sharing Reiki healing with each other, we heard
a gentle knock at the door. It was the man and his friend apol-
ogizing for their tardiness. They curiously strolled inside and
gazed at the tables and practitioners sitting around them.
Looking deeply into my eyes the man asked, "What are you
doing?" My response was, "Reiki Natural Healing—I thought
you were Reiki practitioners."

He laughed and exclaimed, "Oh, I thought you said you
were a Reggae Master!" Clicking his fingers he further indi-
cated, "We came here to dance."

Intrigued by it all they both asked to receive a sample of
Reiki and then were on their way. Later, I was told they had
become Reiki practitioners because of this incident.

Limits Fade Away

Once initiated into Reiki, daily self-treatment and learning to live the Reiki Precepts become our most precious gifts.
As the healing energy assists us to become healthier and happier, life just continues to get better. Old limits we used as

excuses to keep us from moving forward simply fade away and no longer separate us from our true potential.

Before living the life of Reiki I looked at traveling in a completely different way. I was working in the corporate arena and receiving a salary, feeling quite fortunate to have the funds to take vacations to wonderful places. And yet, these periods away were often limited and seemed to take a tremendous amount of planning and juggling of finances to bring to fruition. It was difficult at times to take the job hat off, let go of responsibilities and immediately play for two or three weeks. In the back of my mind lingered the knowledge that I would soon have to return and attempt to get back into my daily occupational routine once more.

After Reiki life has been extremely different from those days. When one truly lives in the flow of Reiki energy it is quite unique. It takes time and the willingness to be flexible, but soon enough one becomes accustomed to living in a harmonious energetic flow. Your work is not really work. Play and fascinating people seem to blend right in with the Reiki schedule. The limits of everyday life take on a new more fluent and pleasant reality. Reiki becomes an aspect of all activities. Sometimes life simply appears to be an ongoing vacation of daily interesting surprises. The more Reiki we receive the more it looks as if no limits in life could be possible.

With Reiki, Dreams Do Come True

Reiki has taken me on incredible journeys and introduced me to charming people from different countries and from different religious and cultural backgrounds. The remarkable fact is that whenever I could keep my mind out of the way, the trips fell into place effortlessly and at the most unexpected yet perfect times. Expenses were always covered in truly unusual ways.

Comedian Mitch Hedberg said, "I'm sick of following my

dreams. I'm just gonna ask where they're going and hook up with 'em later." That is actually what we do with Reiki.

Looking back has brought me the realization that my journeys were ones energetically requested by me at some point in my life. Some even were childhood dreams, an example being a most astonishing trip to Egypt. As a child I would have dreams of riding a camel in Egypt. Although I did grow up in the Arizona desert, we certainly didn't ride camels there!

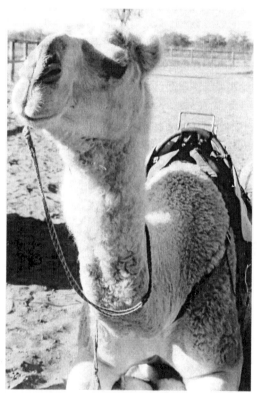

Camel after receiving Reiki

Actually, the first time I rode a camel was not in Egypt. It was during a trip to teach Reiki Classes in Australia. Traveling north in Western Australia our bus stopped at a fun place where we could have a camel ride. I was shocked, never before thinking about those animals living in Australia. The camel owner explained that a great deal of central Australia is desert and camels are valuable for interior travel.

Once on the camel's back, as he was moving up off his knees, I felt so comfortable. Surprisingly, it gave me the impression of being a familiar means of transportation. The same experience happened while riding camels in Egypt. On both occasions, sharing Reiki with them was further valida-tion that all animals enjoy Reiki's healing energy. There is nothing like the expression on a camel's face as they are receiving a Reiki treatment. It actually appears they are smil-ing and in a state of total bliss as they close their eyes and you hear them sigh while watching their entire body begin to relax. It is really exciting to witness!

Another story of how Reiki shows us there are no limits began when a boyfriend invited me to go to Minnesota for Christmas to experience snow and meet his family. Being that I grew up in Arizona decorating saguaro cacti and having out-door barbecues around the swimming pool for Christmas, going somewhere that was very cold didn't really excite me and still doesn't. He offered his assurance that it wouldn't be an issue. He suggested we stop and visit my two daughters and family on the trip, knowing that this was an offer I would-n't refuse. Feeling Reiki's guidance, I accepted the invitation.

The real illustration of no limits began shortly after he pur-chased the airline tickets. The phone rang and it was a friend who excitedly shared with me that I had been invited to join a group of healers who were going to Egypt to perform cere-mony in the Great Pyramid. She explained the new energies being funneled through the pyramid will assist to release the chains of limitation presently being experienced. Masters were being called to help facilitate this energetic flow.

I told her it all sounded lovely, however I had plans to travel just a few days after that event so it was not possible for me to attend. I slept very little that night because my heart really wanted to go to Egypt, not Minnesota!

A few days later, just as I was starting to feel better about not going, the phone rang. This time it was a man handling travel arrangements for the group. He explained that a Reiki person I knew had purchased a ticket and then couldn't go and wanted to offer it to me for a very low price. The ticket departure was from New York City. I explained again about my prior commitment, the fact I would need to come from Hawaii, and that it would mean crossing the Pacific Ocean and most of the United States four times within a month.

Oddly enough it didn't seem to make a bit of difference to this person. Reiki quickly started showing me, there are no limits when one works with the flow of the energy and stops trying to understand and resist its messages.

Well, I went on the excursion and had a marvelous time in Cairo visiting the museum and sharing Reiki in several ancient places. The Great Pyramid ceremony could only be classified as an exquisite Reiki experience of a lifetime. What fun I had riding camels, visiting ancient temples and monuments! While on a seven night deluxe cruise down the Nile River, we stopped and experienced the remains of each of Egypt's seven sacred chakra temples. Immersed in that ancient energy I connected with each temple with a Distant Reiki treatment then, when guided, provided a Reiki Mental treatment for the specific emotional healing that each chakra temple represents. It was an awesome Reiki phenomenon!

The word chakra is a Sanskrit word meaning wheel or disk. Energy centers of the body are called chakras. We have seven major energy centers located along the spinal column and over a hundred others throughout the body. Egypt had seven temples located along the Nile River where initiates would study and learn about each of these spinning wheels of energy and their importance to the body's overall physical and emotional health.

There are healers that provide chakra clearing and balancing sessions. This happens automatically during a Reiki treatment as our innate ability to heal takes the energy to wherever it is needed for healing. There are no limits with Reiki and chakras are important to our health maintenance program.

After this incredible sojourn, I returned home, unpacked and repacked the suitcase for below zero temperatures. I had no idea how cold that could be! Following all the excitement in Egypt, I had an inconceivably out of the ordinary Minnesota Christmas, and was able to visit family in Phoenix and Chicago along the way. Because of many self-Reiki treatments and the loan of the heaviest clothes ever placed on my body, it was all doable and flowed smoothly. There are no limits, except those we create with our mind.

Ask And You Will Receive

Another amazing story that perhaps will help you understand more fully the powerful unlimited flow of Reiki began when a lovely woman named Ingeborg came to Kauai from Berlin for Second Degree training in 1995. She loved the islands and returned several times for visits. We both felt one day I would teach Reiki classes in Berlin. Placing the idea in the back of our minds and not thinking about it for a long time, we knew if it was meant to happen it would. Then we simply sent the idea some Reiki energy to support it's timely development and surrendered to the divine process.

A couple of years later, after picking up mail from the post office box, I decided to stop at a restaurant for something to eat. I selected a table on the outdoor patio, placed the order, and proceeded to sort through my mail. Opening a large envelope from The Reiki Alliance, I pulled out a piece of literature with our sizeable Reiki symbol on it. It became obvious that it drew the attention of the two young ladies seated at a nearby table.

Almost immediately one of them asked if I was a Reiki Master. When I confirmed this they looked disappointed, explaining they had been on the island for two weeks and had been looking for a Reiki Master, and now they found one and were leaving in the morning to return home to Berlin.

Right away I knew what Reiki was up to and was able to enjoy a new level of watching the drama play itself out. When they asked for my business card I suggested they stay in touch and said "You never know when I may be teaching in Europe." They then proceeded to invite me to visit Berlin to teach at their yoga studio. Again, understanding how Reiki works, I told them if it was meant to happen it would come together effortlessly in its own timing.

Not long after my encounter with the ladies from Berlin I was presenting a Reiki introduction on Kauai when in walked Vicky from Luxembourg. Staying after the presentation, she proceeded to ask several questions about my background and Reiki Master training. In due course I accepted her as a Reiki Master Candidate and her minimum of one year training was underway.

We worked together on Kauai for a few weeks before she returned home to New York. A few months later, Vicky was moving right along with her training when I received an invitation to attend the yearly Reiki Alliance conference. This year it was being held in Germany. Vicky speaks five languages and organized classes in Europe as part of her training. While providing the service of a translator, she repeated each word I said in the classes which assisted her on a deeper level to understand the teaching formula.

Impressed once again by Reiki, I watched the energetic dots starting to connect as plans effortlessly came together for this trip. After sending an email to Sabine and Rachel, the two young women I had met in the restaurant, and with support from Ingeborg, my student residing in Berlin, they proceeded to bring together a class. It was surprising how I associated so easily with the energy of the city and her people.

The class included East and West Berliners and was educational on many levels for all. Ingeborg reviewed the class. Her mother also attended the class, making it an even more special occasion.

A year later Sabine returned to Kauai for her Second Degree training and during the visit she met the man that would become her husband. During her next visit I performed their wedding ceremony. I didn't see them until they returned a few years later with two beautiful children.

The Never Ending Reiki Excursions

London is one of my favorite cities, so I knew Reiki wouldn't take me as close as Berlin and not include it. Another Reiki Master extended an invitation to stay in her home while she brought the people together for my classes. She was a splendid hostess and organizer.

This same journey also took me on to Amsterdam where Vicky and I attended a Dutch Reiki Gathering where little English was spoken. It was miraculous how much I could piece together from attending other Reiki activities with no knowledge of the Dutch language. Vicky helped whenever she could without causing too much disturbance.

It was during this event that I learned about using a living Reiki table. I was so excited to find out about it! There were not enough Reiki tables for everyone to share Reiki at the event, so a practitioner spoke up and suggested we use the "living Reiki tables." It was so clever. Three or four chairs were placed facing each other, depending on the length of the receiver, with one chair positioned at the head. The Reiki practitioners filled the chairs and interlocked their knees together with the person across from them.

The receiver sat at the end of the living table and rested back on the legs as they were lifted until their head was in the lap of the person sitting at the other end. The practitioner receiving Reiki was as light as a heavy feather when everyone lifted together to move the receiver off the living table. The experience was splendid. It was like being in a Reiki cocoon. We were not only receiving Reiki from everyone's hands but from their legs and bodies too. The husband and wife Reiki Masters that were giving to my upper body were blind, and the tenderness of their touch was truly memorable. It warms my Reiki heart now just thinking of it.

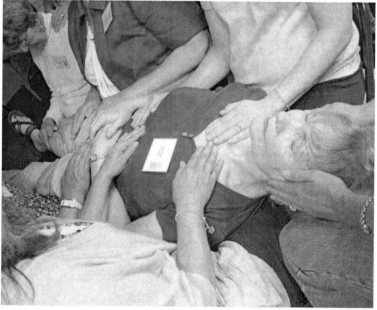

A living Reiki table

Another great adventure was spent in Amsterdam with Tiny, another Alliance Master. As I explored the city it was a new experience for me to see people getting in their boat, just as I would get in my car, to go somewhere.

Once when we were out and about, my eyes caught sight

of a beautiful Reiki magazine and I immediately felt its energy deeply touching my spirit. Walking over to take a closer look, however, was a bit disappointing. It was printed in Dutch, oh well.

I was soon off on the next Reiki escapade when a Reiki Master couple named Simon and Ellen extended an invitation for me to spend a few days with them in Krabbendijke in the southern part of the Netherlands. It was great to take the train there, viewing the lovely countryside along the way, and to share Reiki treatments with them and their students while listening to Simon's healing music flowing peacefully throughout the room.

Later I met Vicky back in Amsterdam and we decided to take a side journey to visit Turkey and Greece. It was fun and relaxing sitting back and playing tourist while enjoying tours of these two countries.

After three months of treatments and trainings, Reiki Gatherings and conferences, it was time to complete the circle and return to Luxembourg to teach a Second Degree class.

Before the Reiki Alliance conference and my class in Berlin, Vicky had organized her first classes during her Master training in and around her hometown in Luxembourg. What a joy it was to initiate her family, friends and new people we hadn't met, while establishing a solid support system to assist her to move into her life as a Reiki Master. Our European tour started and eventually ended in her beautiful country of Luxembourg. I now fully understood her deep love for her country and its friendly people, and really felt quite honored to be her Reiki Master. Vicky's cousin Gerthy and Fernand were our most gracious host and hostess as they continued to welcome us into their home.

After the training Gerthy and I rode a train to Paris where we met and stayed with a friend I had shared a room with on the ship going down the Nile in Egypt. Christmas is her name.

Three healers radiating out powerful energy caused quite a stir while driving around Paris in her brand new convertible automobile with the top down.

Gerthy later took me by train to Vienna, another city I had always wanted to explore. She had friends living there that were away on holiday and invited us to stay in their residence while they were gone. It was fun sharing Reiki and riding around the city in the Fiaker (horse and carriage), a romantic means of transport which in a typically Viennese fashion refuses to die. As Paul Hörbiger put it "Anyone can become a coachman, but only in Vienna can you ride a Fiaker."

After three months of exciting Reiki adventures, Kauai was calling me home again. The Reiki circle of Europe was complete.

Heeding the Call

It seems as we do self-treatments, give and receive full treatments and initiate other people, our energy intensity continues to increase and come into its next level of balance and fullness. Along with this gift arrives another level of healing responsibilities we are asked to share in new situations. When in the flow of this energy, you don't think about not going when you feel called.

The Mexican Riviera cruise was an example. When I received an invitation to attend the 100th birthday party for Gladys Iris Clark, a healer from Sedona, Arizona, I had other financial obligations and yet followed my heart by taking most of the funds available and making a commitment to be there. This was another time I felt Reiki had a need and enticed me to attend, continually testing the idea of not having limits in my life.

Connecting for a few days on a cruise ship with several healers from around the globe is curative within itself. As healing treatments were exchanged, the energy of the cruise escalated and continued to grow. The birthday party took us to Mazatlan, Puerto Vallarta and Cabo San Lucas. In each port they knew our birthday girl and had a Mexican celebration with birthday cake. Many knew Gladys Iris Clark the world over for her healing abilities, spiritual wisdom and experience. At the age of 94 she wrote a book, Forever Young: How to Attain Longevity. The trip couldn't have been better until we started the return voyage to Los Angeles.

The waves were rough and several people including my roommate were experiencing sea sickness. Thank goodness for Reiki! It was the only thing that kept me from literally losing it. In order to sleep it was necessary to keep sending Reiki to my roommate and myself. The second day was worse. I was called to the ship's lobby where several people, including pregnant women, were laying on the floor. Some had been sick most of the night and were concerned about the babies they were carrying. They had taken medication with little relief and didn't want to take more. The ship's doctor asked if I would administer Reiki Natural Healing.

After explaining that it works with all levels of healing—body, mind and spirit—I went from one grateful individual to the next with astounding results. The cruise ship doctor wrote a report and recommended offering Reiki to be taught to the crew members of their ships, again proving there are no limits in what the system of Reiki called Usui Shiki Ryoho can do.

In 2003 I attended an eventful Reiki Alliance conference in Trimurti, France. Flying into Nice with Diane, a Hawaiian Reiki Master I had recently initiated, we made our way to the conference. It was an exciting seven days connecting with Usui Shiki Ryoho masters from various countries. With so much yummy Reiki energy coming together and being shared, I always feel like I've come full circle with Reiki and am starting the upward spiral again. During the conference it is a daily awe-inspiring custom for masters to come together and share treatments and Reiki stories.

After Reiki hug farewells, Diane and I boarded a train to Rome, Italy, where we both visited the Vatican for the first time. That was quite a site for two Reiki masters from Kauai where the buildings can't be constructed higher then the tallest coconut tree.

Then there was the challenge of telling taxi drivers where we wanted to go. Quickly we noticed that they seemed to understand us better when Reiki was used ahead of time. Ordering meals when we didn't speak Italian became quite an adventure. In a few restaurants where we couldn't locate someone who admitted to speaking English, we simply sent Reiki to the menu, pointed our finger at an entree that seemed to have the most energy and prayed. Obviously we had some out of the ordinary meals that needed to be filled with even more Reiki.

Happily we arrived in Venice where most everyone spoke our language. After sending Reiki and envisioning our accom-modations being on the Grand Canal, we had asked the hotel staff in Rome to book the impossible reservation request. Upon arrival we were again shown that there are no limits with Reiki, as we walked into a hard-to-get room with a lovely balcony overlooking the Grand Canal.

Venice's main thoroughfare is busy with all kinds of boats, but the sleek, black, graceful gondolas are a symbol of the city. After sharing Reiki treatments, exploring Venice by boat and walking along the cobblestone streets shopping and view-ing the sights, we took the train along the entire French Riv-iera to Lourdes. As we took pleasure in sending Reiki to our meals in the dining car, we gazed out at all the incredibly gor-geous sites along the way.

In the Southwest of France at about 1,200 feet above sea level in the foothills of the Pyrenees Mountains is Lourdes, the meeting point of the Seven Valleys of the Lavedan. Upon approaching the healing place above us and seeing the castle, it seemed we were entering a fairytale book. Lourdes became famous February 25, 1858 after a young girl saw a vision of Mother Mary and was told to dig in the soil where she was standing. The young girl followed instructions and healing water appeared. Every year more than 3,500,000 pilgrims, visitors and tourists visit Lourdes hoping to be healed by this water, which has been flowing uninterruptedly.

I drank nothing but this healing water for three days, and I customarily drink a great deal of water. The feeling of aliveness from it appeared to be coming from a cellular level. It was an experience I truly believe people used to feel while eating and drinking food and liquid containing more life force energy before so much commercial processing. It was a similar feeling to the experience after Reiki self-treatment, my total being felt alive, really alive. I enjoyed experimenting with the taste and feel of the water before and after adding Reiki to it. It always seemed more refined after adding even more healing energy.

It was remarkable to see all the wheelchairs lined up in front of the hotels. At certain times each day, volunteers wheel people needing healing down the street lined pathway to the healing waters. Some drink and others are fully submerged in the baths. People arrive with all sorts of containers to fill with healing water and take away with them. Of course we couldn't pass up this opportunity.

At The Reiki Alliance conference participants brought samples of water from a special energy place in their country. We each added our sample to a bowl with the globe of the world floating in the center. Once they were brought together and blended, a representative from each country took a small container of the mixture back to their homeland. Now we were traveling with two samples of highly energized healing water.

Following the sharing of Reiki treatments we boarded the bus to Madrid, Spain. On one level, Reiki must have been watching out for us, because it was a horrible bus ride that would have been even worse if we hadn't had treatments before leaving and while on the journey.

Later, things became more exciting during the plane ride to Lisbon, Portugal. Our two Reiki Master hostesses greeted us there with flowers and smiling Reiki faces. After a tour of their beautiful city of Lisbon they took us to a charming bungalow in Cascais which is now on my list of places to return.

Carla and Cristina had been in contact with me regarding organizing a Reiki program in the Lisbon hospital. We had a meeting of Reiki and medical people to get this plan underway with Christina translating English to Portuguese. These two beautiful young ladies created the Reiki Portugal Organization to assist their community to heal and grow with Reiki Natural Healing. It was magnificent sharing Reiki with them and to enjoy the beach in Cascais. Its gorgeous bay and ocean waves reminded us of Kauai, opihi and all, which made it easier to leave the healing energy of Portugal and our new friends to return to Kauai.

Maui Calls

Maui is another beautiful island located in the Hawaiian island chain. It attracted me when I first moved to Hawaii in 1990 and has been drawing more and more of my interest over the years. Each visit seemed to provide a deeper more intimate connection. At times it created a desire for me to live there and yet I continued to think Kauai would always be my home. But then there came the day I was invited to spend a week on Maui with a dear friend.

While he attended meetings in the afternoons I explored Maui from a new perspective. Students seemed to be drawn to me like a magnet and requested Reiki training, so I con-

nected with the University of Hawaii Maui campus to teach
Reiki Natural Healing in the Continuing Education department in the spring. For several years my classes have been
approved for continuing education credit for nurses and massage therapists, this allows them to provide not only their
patients and clients but also themselves with a deeper healing experience.

After this visit I was invited to return to Maui again a few
months later by another group to teach First Degree training.
Each trip I found myself looking at a few more homes for rent.
The energy was continuing to build. Trusting and surrendering to this Reiki process made me feel as if I was on a ride in
an amusement park not knowing what was around the next
corner.

It was soon April and time again for a mainland U.S.
teaching tour. Returning home to Kauai on a Thursday night
after being away for a month it felt wonderfully relaxing to be
home. The next Sunday I was sending distant Reiki to fill my
home with healing energy when a clear message came that,
after sixteen years on Kauai, it was time to move to Maui.

I have learned to pay close attention to these messages.
After reciting the first Reiki Precept, "Just for today, do not
worry" and remembering there are no limits, I was on a plane
to Maui that next Friday.

By Monday evening, after many magical synchronistic
events, I had rented a beautiful new home, had a new phone
number and made arrangements for utilities, without even
taking a moment to think about what was happening. Continual validations of my actions kept pouring in; from the
beautiful rainbow that greeted me upon arrival in Iao Valley
to the unexpected beach front upgrade to my hotel room.

Other synchronistic connections affirmed the move. During the previous December, I had needed another massage
table for a class I was teaching on Maui. I contacted the hotel

where I was teaching and they provided the name of one of their massage therapists. He was most accommodating and delivered his table to the classroom. We connected and offered to help each other in the future if needed.

Four months later, as I was making the move, I found myself calling him to ask if he knew of a home to rent. He gave me the name and telephone number of his landlord, who had a cottage becoming available.

Months before, while looking for the perfect places for Reiki classes for the Maui Reiki trainings, I was given the name of a lady that had classroom space. She too offered her assistance whenever I was visiting Maui. Calling her to inquire about living space she gave me a name and phone number. Little did I know at the time both new friends had supplied the same contact information. One was a cellular phone and the other a landline number.

After arriving on the property I met a woman living in another house there. During our conversation, I learned she is not only the mother of someone I knew on Kauai, but also that her daughter had given me a hat that her mom had left behind. I had been wearing a hat that once belonged to this lady I had just met and who was about to become my neighbor.

Curiosity kicked in as I wondered what other housing opportunities might be available. Checking the local newspaper and a few rental agents provided more validation that when connected to Reiki there are no limits and that I was truly divinely protected. Looking at other housing available was a bit of a frightening experience. Nothing compared to the little cottage up on the hillside with ocean views from each room. As I connected with other places that were becoming available, I was told that my name would be added to a waiting list, or it would be open to view at 10 a.m. on Saturday and would go to the first person to sign the lease.

There was no doubt this is where I needed to be living. The move to Maui occurred in May, three days before the Reiki class at the University I had scheduled back in October. Little did I know at that time I would be a Maui resident while teaching this class.

As students were introducing themselves I mentioned my writing project. Out of the twelve students one announced she was a writer, another an illustrator and a third said her mother was a publisher. After class the writer asked if I would consider being interviewed for an article about my move to Maui for the Maui Weekly newspaper. By attending the class she was able to create a detailed story and include energetic material not available any other way. It was just the energy needed to introduce me to the Maui community and start a new client base.

Reiki Growth Challenges Continue

I offer these stories as an example of living in the flow and not questioning where the energy is taking you. Clues are provided for us along the way. The important thing is to learn to pay attention and hear these messages. After Reiki training, we quickly learn that the thinking mind often creates limits for us in our life.

When I excitedly shared the news of moving to Maui, it was amazing to note all the different reactions. Those that were not so connected with the energy flow of life questioned how I would survive leaving behind sixteen years of clients, students and friends. Knowing my rent had doubled, with no prospects at all of funds coming in to cover the increased obligation, they were genuinely concerned.

For a quick flash my mind started to get involved; but I was happy to hear myself explain that those particulars were not my concern. When the energy directs me, it handles all the details. Kauai clients that understood how Reiki energy works were excited about the new experience of receiving their series of treatments from a distance. Students were happy to know there was a new place in the islands to visit and share Reiki. Others looked at it simply as an expansion of our Kauai Reiki community.

Not long after the 20-foot container had been unloaded on Maui and all my worldly treasures were unboxed and in their proper place, I settled in and was starting to relax enjoying the incredibly beautiful sunsets from my lanai. The landlord, a new mainland owner, then informed me that he wanted to do some construction on the home I had just settled into, stating he would terminate the six-month lease if I wanted to move. As any Reiki Master would do, I sent Reiki to the situation asking, "What is this all about?"

Whenever I'm not yet to know the divine reason behind something, the energy always guides me to the first Reiki Precept, "Just for today, do not worry."

After several years of living the life of a full-time Reiki Master, experience has proven that whatever surprises are waiting they are always better than what was left behind. Reiki teaches us to live in the now enjoying each moment to its fullest. Trusting and surrendering to the divine plan shows us there are no limits. So why get in the way and muddle things up because we think we know how life is supposed to be? The second Maui home came to me as effortlessly as the first. The mother of the friend from Kauai sent me to a larger, more private home less than a mile away, with even better ocean views from each room.

Once I surrendered to the process and remembered I had no limits with Reiki, new Maui friends arrived and handled most of the move for me.

Removing perceived limits requires learning to let go of the analytical mind and simply allowing the heart, which knows on a deeper level, to provide direction. In the beginning, as the mind refuses to surrender, it can be difficult. It is similar to disciplining a young child or training an animal. You simply can't give in or the process will need to start all over again.

The more we learn not to pay attention to the doubts and fears of the mind and follow our heart's guidance, the easier and more wonderfully life's details simply fall into their proper place.

The purpose of these stories is to share with you how magically life can unfold when we allow it to, trusting that there are no limits. The more we keep this connection to our energetic flow, the more the word freedom continues to take on a new, more personally, expanded meaning.

Reiki gives us permission to know who we are.

*When the steps of our journey have led us to living
a life of Reiki there is but one word left to discover:
Freedom.*

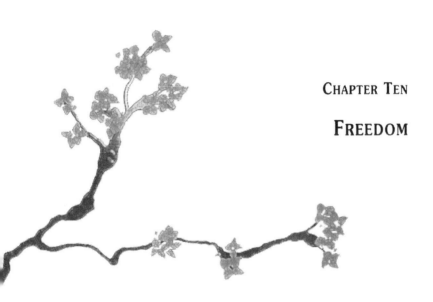

CHAPTER TEN

FREEDOM

The ultimate step in the Reiki growth process is Freedom. We all seem to be searching for Freedom in one form or another—and living the life of Reiki awakens a Freedom within us like no other.

By understanding the nature of energy in our lives and learning about the lineage of Usui Shiki Ryoho (Usui System of Reiki); by receiving treatments and training, using the precepts and practicing self-treatment and treatments for other people, and by handling the flow of things like money, trust and life changes that come to us—we begin to live a life without limits and therefore begin to achieve true Freedom.

It is helpful to understand that Freedom is not a final destination, but an exciting spiraling journey that continues to fulfill us on the deepest levels of our being. Sometimes I envision it as the sleeping Kundalini; the coiled serpent energy

Hindu tradition tells us will awaken as we do and move up our spine to activate each chakra (seven major energy centers) until it reaches the top of the head and is then released, setting our energies and us free.

And in Reiki, like life in general, Freedom always seems to go back to this basic fact: The more we heal ourselves on all levels of body, mind and spirit, the more feelings of Freedom are naturally experienced. What surprises most of us is that with Reiki healing happens regardless of whether or not we know we need it and we don't even have to believe in it for it to work!

Complete Healing Modality

There is so much more to healing than most of us have even started to consider. And before it is possible to experience true inner and outer Freedom, each of us needs to go through various types of emotional healing.

During Reiki treatments people sometimes report seeing colors and know from experience that these relate to the various types of emotions surfacing for healing. When the colors are seen we realize that Reiki energy is most likely bringing healing to the energy center in our body related to that color.

Because Reiki's healing energy automatically goes to where the healing is most needed, it takes care of these emotions as a natural part of treatment. It requires no special effort from the practitioner for chakra clearing or alignment.

Information about the chakras is not part of Reiki classroom teachings. I am presenting them here purely as an example of how Reiki energy is a deep, complete healing modality and works at healing beyond where our limited mind may desire or need to go—and because people are often curious if they see colors during Reiki.

Energy Centers Of Our Body

Each energy center is called a chakra and is known to hold the power of specific emotions and important aspects of our healing process. Each chakra has a color related to the musical vibration of the energy concentrated there. When the chakras are aligned, clear and spinning freely, we experience an incredible sense of Freedom from the mundane difficulties of life. To further explain, here are some examples of the colors and healing properties related to each of our spinning energy centers.

Number One resides near the base of our spine and relates to the color red. It is usually seen during Reiki treatments when the emotions of anger and insecurity we have been storing within are being healed. This energy center helps us and all we do to become more grounded. Through our roots we gain nourishment, power, stability and growth. Without this connection we are separated from nature, from our source. Cut off, we are easily manipulated.

Number Two is located just below our navel and is the color orange. When someone happens to see the color orange during a Reiki treatment it normally means the energy is working to heal energetic blocks around the issue of sexuality and pleasure. This center helps us to obtain better material comfort. Sexuality is a resolution and celebration of our differences; it connects what separates us, or makes us feel alone. Quite simply none of us would be here without it!

Number Three can be found just above the navel and its color is yellow. It is our power center and sometimes called the seat of our emotions. Issues of power, control and personal Freedom surface during this healing. It asks us to refine our concept of power to be one that enhances, empowers, strengthens and develops.

Number Four is the heart center and is usually seen as a beautiful green, or sometimes it can appear as the color pink. This is known as the central point of the Chakra System. It is our energetic core, the inner spirit that unites all the other forces above and below, within and without. Above we have our abstract spirit and mental realms; below we have our "worldly" chakras. When we have healed issues from the lower chakras we are truly on our way to lasting health, well-being and more juicy Freedom! The fourth chakra's job is to integrate and balance the realms of mind and body bringing us a sense of wholeness and peace. When in balance we feel "at home" with ourselves and our world.

Number Five tells us that now we need to start communicating what the lower chakra lessons have taught us. The fifth chakra is located in the throat region. Its color is blue. It is our gateway to health, consciousness and Freedom. From the moment we cry out as a new born child we are starting to express this energy of communication. This is the center of sound, vibration and self-expression. It is the realm of consciousness that controls, creates, transmits and receives communication, both within ourselves and between each other.

Number Six is the brow chakra, an energy located in the center of the head right behind the forehead. Its color is indigo and it is associated with what some call the third eye. As our physical eyes are tools of perception for the brain, the energy called the third eye can be thought of as our psychic perception floating between the two physical eyes. Some consider it our spiritual center.

Number Seven is known as the crown chakra because it crowns the whole system. Its color is violet and it symbolizes being in our highest state of harmony, regal and glorified while organically ruling everything within instead of it ruling us. We are in our natural state of the all-encompassing bounty of expanded consciousness. Our internal house has been cleaned. We have reconnected with the energy from whence we came.

This brings us to the end of our journey of the seven major chakras. We actually have many more of these spinning energy centers connected with our physical body, including the soles of our feet and the palms of our hands. If needed, Reiki energy will routinely take care of their healing because the energy centers are an important part of who we are.

Just as we can look at the body's other systems like the circulatory or digestive system, the energetic chakra system is one of the basic building blocks of our being. For many people Reiki is a way to connect deeper with the energetic reality of themselves. This also extends into the environment as we begin to recognize our connection to the energetic qualities of nature and everything around us.

Energy Centers Of The Land

Throughout the years of providing treatments, teaching Reiki, and playing on the various Hawaiian Islands and around the globe, it has been fascinating to discover the chakras (energy systems) of the land and how they affect us. In Hawaii, for example, each of our seven islands going right up the chain carries similar energies to the seven ancient chakra healing temples in Egypt, the ones mentioned in the preceding chapter.

It is important to be aware of these energies where you live and how they may be affecting your own energy, and visa-versa. With Reiki, intentionally or not, we continually move forward to heal all levels of our being, which in turn effects the healing of all things in our environment and beyond.

Reiki gives us a fast, direct connection to the healing source of our lives. Similar to the teachings of various religions, we are all trying to get to the same place—back home to reconnect with the energy from whence we came.

With Reiki's gentle, and sometimes not so gentle, push

and guidance, we are constantly discovering how to get there and to become healthier, happier individuals.

Reiki Precepts Are A Tool To Heal The Mind

Reiki practitioners are also blessed to have the Reiki Precepts which keep us in the now. Life becomes easier and more enjoyable as we repeatedly allow the wise words of the Precepts to teach us. Emotionally on very deep levels they release stress, anxiety and unhealthy habits. If we just for today do not worry or anger, that alone gives us back priceless energy to play with. By honoring our parents, teachers and elders, earning our living honestly, and showing gratitude to every living thing, our understanding of how truly blessed we are continues to grow and lift us higher and higher.

It is a complete and lasting package supported by Reiki energy for healing our thoughts, while thoroughly blending with other aspects of healing to create an all around wellness program. Insecurities drop away as we step into that unbeatable power of staying connected to our energetic source, reaping us unending benefits and Freedom.

How do you feel at night when you are ready for sleep and when you awake in the morning? Imagine adding to the routine of preparing for the night's rest and for your new day, the added benefit of relaxing to the max by supplying your body with healing energy.

This can be done after Reiki initiations by simply placing your hands on the body. Contact starts the flow of healing energy to quiet the mind and calm the body for quality sleep time. In the morning instead of feeling sluggish and wondering how you will make it through the day, relying on the caffeine from coffee or tea, allow Reiki to supply a healthier energy for you.

Plus, after recalling the Precepts, your mind is relaxed and free of worry and anger, you are ready to honor everyone you come in contact with as a teacher. It becomes a brilliant process to earn your living honestly and show gratitude to every living thing.

There may even be mornings when you get to the point of stretching your arms out to the heavens and asking, "What fascinations are waiting to unfold for me today?" I truly believe this is the way we were intended to have pleasure in life. And when we take the hand of Reiki, we are shown step-by-step how each day we can encounter more of this type of unique Freedom.

Freedom In Action

Sometimes there are things in life we just must do. We don't know why and actually it doesn't seem to matter why, we just do it and it feels right. Afterwards there is often a real awareness of elation and newly blossomed independence bubbling up like a fountain from within. An inner driving force that is stronger then the logical thinking mind is in the driver's seat.

During these times, while we're in the middle of an activity, we may find ourselves realizing and then asking ourselves, "Why am I doing this?" When this happens, there is a clear understanding that we are connected with the flow. Energy is guiding us unerringly onward to more Freedom in all areas of our life. There is a powerful awareness present at that moment. If we want to know anything, all we need to do is ask, feel it and it will be the correct answer.

Possibly this is a real "aha" moment as we discover we've finally found inside ourselves this connection that we have been searching for somewhere outside ourselves. A new sense of Freedom comes over us and it feels absolutely great!

Something at that moment may even be telling us: Wow, it actually takes much less effort to know when we are really in the flow! Can life actually be this easy? We start to savor the taste of more Freedom coming to us as we recognize that our previous freewill choices have created each and every one of our experiences, whether we like it or not.

Next comes an absolute knowing that once we have the answers from our inner voice they are of little use unless applied. At this point, with our awareness activated, we set out to solve the mystery of how to start consistently applying our new wisdom and create a life truly worth living. This is often when Reiki will find and assist those that are really serious about their forward movement. Without a shadow of a doubt, when we trust and surrender to whatever it takes to enjoy Freedom to its fullest, Reiki guides us to proceed in a protected way. That's right, protected. When we are connected to the source of all things what could possibly provide us with more protection?

Reiki's energy will certainly take us to our limits and each time it will push us a little further in our healing, but it is never more than we are capable of handling. Healing energy starts releasing blocked energy from all levels of our being; physical, emotional, spiritual and mental. We are organically directed towards our natural flow.

As this occurs, magical synchronicities become common experiences. They bring an extra level of assurance for easily applying our inner-knowing that we are on the right track to everyday happenings. For example, the person we need to talk to is standing in line right beside us at the grocery market. Or we are planning to travel and the one location of interest is offering a special discount. Or the energy of a certain restaurant has been calling us to visit, feeling we simply must check it out, and a friend sends a gift certificate to dine there.

These are examples of living in the flow of life's energies while reaping the benefits of our thought creations returning to us. While being in this flow, considering the possibility of any kind of limits is out of the question. All that is likely is the next gift from the universe, the source of everything. Our contribution is to simply do Reiki and stay out of the way. This is Freedom like no other!

What Does The Word Freedom Mean To You?

If you were asked what your existence would be like if you were given the reward of Freedom, what would you envision for your life?

Webster's Collegiate Dictionary defines the word Freedom as: 1) The quality or state of being free 2) The absence of necessity, coercion, or constraint in choice or action.

It is an easy out to blame society and say, "Freedom isn't possible in today's world." But, guess what? It is not only possible; it is waiting patiently for our finding! Independence comes in many forms. What does it conjure up for you? Not getting up in the morning at a certain time to go to work. Having unlimited financial Freedom or living in good mental and physical health. Perhaps we desire to enjoy the ideal lover, family and friends. All is possible!

It seems we are always searching outside ourselves for the answers. Life would be so perfect if…I only had this answer or knew when such and such would happen, or had a new car, house, job, lover, and then my life would be different. I could relax and enjoy myself.

Security is not about having things; it's about handling things. We learn to answer all what-ifs with an attitude of gratitude. I can handle any situation now in a loving, positive way. No need to carry it into the future. After all, if we were taking no risks, we wouldn't be enjoying many of the goodies life has waiting for us. What a waste!

A friend once shared with me a wise quote from John Lennon, "Life is what happens to you while you are busy making other plans." Remember, if the moment you are experiencing is not beautiful—then recreate it. We all have freewill to some degree no matter what our personal circumstances happen to be. The trick is to first admit it, learn to understand it, and then use it. Do you normally focus on all the reasons why you can't do the things you want, or do you focus on all the reasons why you can? The choice is ours and our life is a reflection of our choices. It's that simple!

Divine Timing For Internal Freedom

When one practices Reiki and enjoys the benefits of living a life supported by healing energy, there is a genuine appreciation of the value of divine timing. As a Reiki Master who enjoys living the life of Reiki, I have to continually release the expectations and timing of my goals to the energy of life. Whenever I can do that, the immense Freedom that overcomes me is beyond any goal or limited words to express it.

Those goals unfailingly become desires firmly placed in the energetic field to manifest in their Divine Order. No longer is there a need to feel the weight of responsibility for them. Most importantly is the Freedom this allows to enjoy other energies of life while they are incubating.

Hawaiian Rules tell us that "Goals are deceptive. The unaimed arrow never misses." Personally I like to make my desires known, release them, and then wait for them or something better to manifest.

We may be looking for internal Freedom, perhaps simply as a way to quiet those busy thoughts that bind us. I have met physically disabled individuals that are confident and satisfied that they have no limits in the races they can win and the travels they can take in their mind. Others in the best of physical health may not be able to find that internal peaceful place.

Once we are aware that we have inner restrictions (in Reiki we call them blocked energy) we start to recognize that we have the power to remove them. As we consciously work with our total healing process one step at a time, we move closer to our true potential. It is not a matter of possibility; the cosmic trick is how much we are willing to commit to this process. The pathway to Freedom is paved by an indisputable desire and commitment.

Where Is The True Me?

When my daughter Tammi was a young girl in grade school she said something that left a lasting impression to assist with my healing process. During the afternoon while housecleaning together, I had answered the telephone about three times. After the third phone call, I will never forget her looking up at me with those big blue innocent eyes and simply saying, "Mommy why do you sound so different when you talk to different people?"

Reflecting on the recent conversations was a real eye-opener. My words, volume and tone of voice were extremely diverse during each call. I had to look within and search for answers as to why with some people there was such an effort to impress and others almost rudeness was present. None of the conversations seemed to reflect my true personality.

After receiving this awareness I was on a quest to find out who and where the real me was located. Little did I know how long I would be on that quest. I started to discover piece by piece the real me that had been hidden away for such a long time.

How many masks are you wearing? Once our energy comes into balance, and our true personality shines through, the masks can be safely thrown away. It is so awakening and stimulating to actually meet our true self and experience such relief and Freedom by just naturally being who we truly are, while at the same time understanding it is okay and the way it is really meant to be.

Do you ever feel you have an inventory of invisible masks that can be slipped on and off without even being aware you are doing it? You know, you are one person at work, another at the gym, someone else when you are with certain friends and on and on. Ask yourself: Can I wear the same mask for everyone I have contact with in my environment? One day will it be safe to take them off, discard them and wear no mask, continually revealing my true self?

Not until Reiki came into my life did this start to happen for me. Reiki kept showing me more and more masks that were false security items I was carrying around, until the true me was finally found and brought forth to shine its light.

Some days we may ask, "Who am I really and why am I here?" What is the purpose of all of this drama? Is life really meant to be so difficult?

Recently I've been hearing these pleas for understanding more frequently from clients, students and friends.

This insight becomes clearer as we persistently make a conscious effort to find the enjoyment and appreciation that are a part of each precious moment. As we learn to trust in the Divine Order of things and live in the now, continually striving to live the Reiki Precepts, we realize more fully that the present moment is actually all we ever have anyway. It is important to remember that nothing ever really happened in the past or the future, it happened in the now.

Yes our past did create who we are today but we have already lived those moments. If we aren't careful, the illusions of our identification with the past can provide excuses to why things couldn't be the way we would really like them right now. As Reiki healing guides us to leave the past behind, we live more fully in the moment watching limitation after limitation gently, and sometimes not so gently, melt away. Suddenly, everything feels alive and real reflecting a new, different, distinctive kind of nourishing energy. This allows us to richly be in the present, a place where the past ceases to have any power to keep us from this precious moment now. We simply have no need to live there anymore.

Each day, as the energetic flow of life guides us forward to new adventures, it becomes easier to surrender—with no need to get in the way or try to control the future. No expectations, no disappointments.

Many dreams are cast aside because of public opinion and tradition. Ambitions have been postponed for unnecessary reasons. Lives have been lived for a tomorrow which never came. Ask yourself now, "If I only had a short while to live, what would I be doing right now?" Don't dwell on the fear, but consider your opportunities. Then do it! Just do it! Why not take pleasure in every moment of life now? You deserve it!

We can become masters of our lives if we just make our desires known and then release them—providing the Freedom for their return or something better to come to us. Why waste time in fantasy worlds of past and future or be a puppet controlled by society's influences? Step into your new life. Find out who you really are.

It is your birthright to be healthy and happy, generating love in whatever manner that may take for you.

Observe each habitual tendency to want to slip back to the old ways that created limitation. Then decide what is most important and will bring the most joy. As we switch focus and find the excitement of each moment, each heartbeat, true appreciation and enjoyment starts to occur more frequently. Soon they become a new exciting way of life. We have found Freedom! Usui Shiki Ryoho provides a proven tool to keep us connected to our source, thusly living wholly every valuable moment.

As The Healing Adventure Continues

Recently I moved to a thrilling new level of living in Freedom's bliss. While accomplishing mundane tasks, I was unexpectedly overcome with the feeling of joy! Several days passed and I found myself saying, "The last few days have been perfect. I don't know how I could have made them any better." Excitement and humble gratitude moved throughout my being as the realization became clear. I don't need anything to be happy. I feel fulfilled. It truly is possible. What a divine gift!

One evening after a Reiki class in Littleton, Colorado, some of the students and I went to dinner at a Chinese restaurant. Following our meal we each opened and read out loud the message tucked inside our fortune cookie. As I was reading mine we all started to laugh. I kept it as a helpful reminder. It read, "You are the master of every situation."

This is true! We really have that ability. Reiki provides an important means to discover mastery leading to Freedom from the drama we encounter in our everyday lives. As healing takes place inside, the benefits happen outside. There is simply no other way. Along with this comes an awareness of our own mastery and how to express it honestly.

A beautiful Hawaiian family of ten on Kauai felt guided and asked for Reiki training, they trusted this was something they all needed to do together. They had seen and experienced wonderful results through treatments and commented that they now wanted the Freedom to provide Reiki for themselves and each other. Young children, their parents and grandparents were all present.

Soon after the training, a family member became ill with cancer and was told she had only a short while to live. The family was eternally grateful for the choices Reiki Natural Healing provided for them during a painful, stressful time. They not only were able to provide comfort for the pain from the disease, but the energy also assisted their loved one with the fear of passing. In addition, as the end of life came for their loved one, it made the process easier for them because they could share healing energy with each other.

Looking back at our lives it is clear that a quest for Freedom from something or another was always present. From the time of conception we are given the gift of an opportunity to grow into a baby. Disconnection from mother offers a new kind of Freedom.

Then there were all the different stages of growth and development; the lack of restrictions when we learn to crawl, then to walk, ride a bike, escape the home limits and attend school. The liberties to drive a car, date, marry and have children, then grandchildren. Going into the job market with a specialty profession continues to provide a new sense of independence.

Then before we know it we think retirement is what will really bring us Freedom. But oftentimes, soon after retirement, those health problems we have collected over the years start to surface along with a realization that maybe through dying and returning to the source from which we came provides the only true Freedom.

We can start now, this very second, to live completely. In each moment we can eternalize the stages of Freedom and know they are an important element of who we are. We can truly understand that these Freedoms are a vital aspect of uniting body, mind and spirit and guide us towards greater levels of self-actualization and joy.

How Can Spirit Alter Our Quality Of Life?

We each have a mind, body and spirit. We know a lot about our bodies and our minds, but how many of us know about our spirit? Spirit is the source of our highest wisdom and truth. You may know it as higher self, intuition, place of peace, hunch, inner voice/guidance, inspiration or experience of the presence of God within.

Our mind chatters constantly. It wants to control our consciousness. The quality of many people's lives and the problems we face in the world today are a result of our disconnection from spirit. In order to get to spirit, we need to quiet the mind. Reiki Natural Healing lovingly assists with this process. We soon learn to accept our Freedom of choice and remind ourselves that peace does not mean to be in a place where there is no noise, trouble or hard work. It means to be in the midst of those things, to stay connected to our source and remain calm and joyful in our heart.

A dear friend and Reiki practitioner once told me that spirit had given him the spiritual name Eagle Heart to give to me. I was told as I walked the sacred path of life my name would reveal its meaning to me.

Later a Hopi elder further explained:

"Your name Eagle Heart in Hopi is Kwahu
Unungwa, heart of the eagle is a healer of
hearts who carries the Father's Power within
her breast. Eagle is the protector and
guardian of Tis, all that is above, and is our
messenger to the Father. To be of the
Father's heart is very powerful. It means you
have the ability to call upon the Father's
strength for healing and spiritual gifts
needed in your life and in the life of others.
It is represented by the spotted eagle, one of
many colors like the rainbow or colors of
ears of corn; as Great Spirit "Tawa" and
Earth Mother's children are all colors and
none are above the others, only in responsibility as they act with true hearts. As I know
that the Reiki energies are from the Father
your name is perfect for you."

There were times when the name appears to make known

more and more hidden significance. Recently, I came to see clearly the truth it holds for me at this time. The eagle represents a strong sense of Freedom as it glides so gracefully and yet powerfully above the mundane trivia of life's many challenges, and yet there are times when it needs to connect with them in order to sustain itself in the physical.

Major Global Changes

My heart is full of love for this planet and all of her people. I give thanks to Reiki for its support, love and guidance to find unerring Freedom in a place where misleading concepts seem to be the way of existence and complications of living have become a real challenge.

Going back in history we find this has often been the case when it is time for major global change. It is indeed a difficult and sometimes threatening time for all of us. It is also an astonishing opportunity for awareness and growth if we choose to accept it that way.

Millions of people all over the world are seeking to transform and improve their lives. They are now painfully aware that the answers for a changed world are not coming from sources outside themselves. The answers lie within.

Today we are moving away from a society that accepted the x-ray, but refused to believe that human vision can see beneath the skin. It accepted the telephone, and yet denied word awareness beyond the range of the human ear. We accomplished travel to outer space, and yet wouldn't accept the ability of the mind to travel outside the limits of the body. Our surgeons accomplished amazing things with a scalpel and yet denied miracles achieved by human beings administering healing energy.

This is no longer the case today, as those limited thoughts are a thing of the past. Remarkable opportunities for progress are presenting themselves daily. Reiki Natural Healing is among the leading modalities for today's new health care vision of positive progress, helping to heal global changes affecting our planet, ourselves and future generations.

The incredibly gentle practice of Reiki healing adds another dimension to both our personal and professional life. Continually it reminds us to connect with the inner source of wholeness that stands ready to work miracles by just a tender placement of hands. Every new day is a lesson in the adage that the transformation of the world we see begins with the transformation of how we see ourselves.

The ability to understand and love everyone and everything in our lives begins with understanding and loving ourselves. This provides a kind of personal road map for achieving spiritual clarity that can make the transformation of inner attitude to improve outer reality. Reiki is a Divine Gift whose time has come!

More Understanding

As you began reading this book, the meaning of certain words such as energy or life force may not have been clear to you at first. Hopefully by now you have received deeper understanding and clarity about how important this transformative power really is to your personal Freedom. Each chapter has taken you on a journey to the next stage of development in the never-ending quest for healing all aspects of your being.

Perhaps Reiki practitioners understand more fully the value in trusting Reiki and have surrendered deeper to its guidance, resulting in our life becoming simpler, more fun and exciting as we find where the energy of life wants to take us.

Learning to act on guidance while trusting the information received brings a comforting feeling of Freedom. Knowing that Reiki is a lasting lifelong connection continually awakening in us other healing gifts brings an indescribable sense of security. As we learn from wonderful experiences to trust, we just naturally have faith in the inexhaustible source of energy within ourselves.

May this story of my search for healing with Reiki's guidance be helpful to you in seeking health and happiness by reducing conflict, anger, confusion and stress in your life.

When I began my investigation of understanding the spiritual aspect of my nature, the missing pieces of the puzzle of the human condition began to fall into place. It wasn't easy; it took work, discipline, lots of Reiki, practicing the Reiki Precepts daily and a concentrated effort in unraveling the ancient techniques of Usui Shiki Ryoho. The more I applied Reiki and the knowledge gained by my investigation, the more I found myself, my attitudes, and my perceptions transforming my life into a more positive and peaceful adventure.

I love living the life of a Reiki Master and all the unlimited possibilities it continues to offer. I invite you to connect with your healing ability and receive from Reiki what level of support is perfect for you. The healing journey begins with the first step and it is never too late to take the first or last step to our source of Freedom. The power is in your hands!

Reiki Hands

There's energy within us
That comes from out our hands
A universal energy
Not all can understand.
This radiant source for healing,
A gift from up above,
The Reiki that we share within,
We give to each with love.

by Greg Goodson, Reiki Master
Red Bluff, California

**Millions have benefited from
Reiki Natural Healing, and so can you.**

*A Reiki book would not be complete
without success stories.*

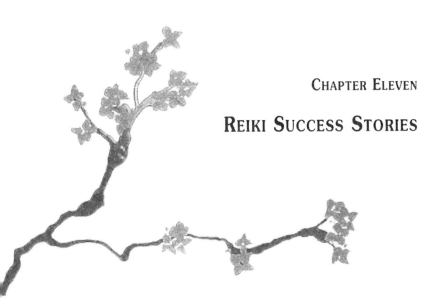

CHAPTER ELEVEN

REIKI SUCCESS STORIES

This collection was compiled from clients, students, colleagues and friends who excitedly shared their experiences. I am grateful to them for taking a few minutes to put their words in writing so that others may understand more fully what is possible with Reiki Natural Healing.

I invite you to continue sending your stories to add to the collection for future editions.

Reiki Lowers Blood Pressure

A few years ago I experienced a heart attack. After my Reiki training and administration of self-treatments, my medication is no longer needed for my heart condition. Reiki has also lowered my blood pressure and helps me to relax.

**Earl
Kauai, Hawaii**

Reiki Heals the Impossible

I learned about Reiki from my wife Jenna who became a First Degree Practitioner and treated me, and I was hooked. I had never felt so relaxed and at peace. Several months later I became a First Degree Reiki Practitioner graduating to Second Degree shortly thereafter all the while I was doing several series of treatments with Reiki Master Shalandra and performing self treatments. The healing that I was blessed to receive was nothing short of extraordinary.

In less than 5 months of treatments my body was virtually healed of all seasonal allergies that I have lived with my whole life. Being able to breathe again when you gasp for air 3 months out of the year for close to 40 years: Priceless.

In addition I have suffered from severe episodes of low back pain for 20 years with a compression fracture and several herniated discs, and I feel like I am very close to putting that behind me for life as well. I've had 2 minor episodes in 5 months when I've been accustomed to a major episode almost every month for 5 years.

Next my wrist. A chronic injury to my right wrist had threatened my career as a Chiropractor to the point of having to quit for over 2 years due to disability. Well I'll tell you that my wrist is even better than my low back. And for the 1st time in my career I have no fear of disability. Plus, because of this healing, Reiki has saved my golf game.

Lastly and most importantly I truly believe that Reiki had saved my marriage. My wife and I came to a new level of understanding, peace, and love that I could not see developing at all without "Our Reiki."

Bless you Reiki you have truly been a gift from the divine!

Dr. Anthony Jayswal
Owner of Healing Hands Chiropractic Of Maui
Lahaina, Hawaii

Reiki Class Brings Major Life Shift

The entire Reiki class was truly an experience. Reiki is a unique way to connect with people you've never met, on a universal energy level. During my self-treatment in class, I felt blocks of energy dispersing down my right leg, like mini explosions in very specific spots. During the first initiation, I felt one of those mini explosions on the right side of my frontal lobe (head), which is where I get one of my headaches. I have had sinus problems for years and they are now clearing up due to the new sinus drainage. My ears have cleared out, also. After receiving Reiki for an hour on the Reiki table in class, I felt shots of energy shoot down my arms like nerve pain, but the shooting was not painful.

My body is detoxing, physically and emotionally. Things have come up for me that I have not dealt with in years, and with the intensity of it all, I am still healing more while I do my self-treatments. Rapid changes are happening and I 'just go with it.' ALSO...I have been falling asleep with my hand on my head, accessing dreams and memories from my childhood I did not know were there. Dreams have been vivid, unlocking and healing subconscious memories.

It has been 14 years that I have subconsciously and habitually been grinding my teeth... I still do it, but not nearly as much, and I am down to two cigarettes a day. I have never been able to cut down on grinding my teeth as I have now. It was so bad my jaw sometimes wouldn't move due to stress and past triggers. I cannot thank you enough for showing me this incredible gift.

I am going to get a journal to start recording these newly found discoveries and answers that have been blocked energy for me for years. Again, thank you, so much Shalandra. The Reiki class was 100 percent worth it and I feel the beginning of a long, healthy, shift in my life.

Trevor
Maui, Hawaii

Diabetes Healed...Becomes Reiki Master

The main purpose for me to take Reiki training was to help control my diabetes. I faithfully practiced Reiki on myself at least three times daily, and within six weeks I had lowered my blood sugar count by almost 100 points, and also my eyes improved so much that I no longer need my glasses to read and sew. After taking Second Degree Reiki I felt even more extra healing power.

I originally took Reiki to use just on myself, and then I found myself sharing this wonderful gift with members of my family and friends. I am now a Reiki Master and enjoy teaching Reiki.

Betty
Denver, Colorado

Cancer Healed

Desi found out she had cancer in February of last year. She was experiencing very itchy skin on her feet, legs and hands. After losing weight she finally went to see a doctor and was diagnosed with cancer in her chest. She began to research alternative ways to heal. People prayed for her, and came up with different drinks and diet plans to try.

Her grandmother passed away from cancer the following month. Her cancer had gone into remission and came back a month later with vengeance. Desi did not want to take chemotherapy because she saw how sick it made her grandmother. And Desi could probably not take care of her baby if she was feeling sick.

When I found out about the situation, I went to her home to see her. She showed me how bad her legs were with scars and explained about the itching on her hands and legs. I told her I was going to take a First Degree Reiki class soon and hopefully that could help.

After taking my class, I saw her several times and gave her Reiki treatments. She was using a chili pepper mixture to rub on her chest. It was actually burning her chest leaving a huge mark. I gave her Reiki there to help with the pain.

Three months later, with all the different treatments and diets, nothing seemed to be helping, and she appeared to be getting worse instead of better. I told her I would soon be taking Second Degree Reiki and would send her treatments. Until I sent her Reiki in June, Desi did not want to take chemotherapy. The first week she stopped everything else and only received distant Reiki every morning. During these treatments she was divinely guided to start chemotherapy as I continued to send her morning Reiki treatments.

Later I went to see her, she was doing okay and had only gotten slightly sick from the therapy and lost only a few strands of her long hair. She said she felt energized every morning and could move around until she got tired in the afternoon. She slowly improved and the itching finally stopped. She was spending more time going to the beach and having fun swimming and riding the jet ski as she acquired a nice suntan. Another cancer patient asked what she did and couldn't believe how she could spend so much time in the sun at the beach. She explained to her about her Reiki treatments. Her progress continued to get better and she slowly was putting on some needed weight in all the right places.

I continued sending Reiki daily. By December, the cancer had decreased from 14 millimeters to 2 millimeters. The scars on her leg were slowly clearing up. She was on a diet of water, veggies, fruits and seafood. Her attitude was good. She was just living life and enjoying every moment. She seemed more relaxed and patient.

At Christmas I let Desi know I was still sending Reiki to her every morning and would continue to send. She was very thankful. In February Desi was clear of cancer! She looked good with all her hair and the right amount of weight. Her legs were almost clear of the scars. There were just a few small ones on her feet. She was in good spirits.

As of April, she is still doing well, as she continues therapy accompanied by my morning Reiki treatments. Her legs are completely healed and she has started dancing hula again. Her family wonders where she is getting all this energy from to do so much without getting tired. By looking at her with that beauty and smile-you would never know that she had gone through such a great ordeal.

Diane
Kauai, Hawaii

Muscle Relaxation, Increased Energy and Mental Clarity

I was first introduced to Reiki two years ago by close friends. My husband was fighting LOU GEHRIG'S DISEASE and we were exploring a variety of healing modalities in particular because there is no cure or treatment for the illness and it is degenerative and terminal in nature. Our friends gave my husband Reiki treatments and he experienced overall relaxation from his muscle contractions and an increase in energy as a result.

As a full-time caregiver for my husband the last three years, I experienced considerable fatigue and learned the importance of taking care of oneself. I explored Reiki healing treatments and completed First Degree training and I have recognized many therapeutic benefits from self-treatments and treatments received by other Reiki Practitioners. In particular, I have experienced less aches and pains from a back injury, which has been troublesome over the last few years. Also, I have an increase in energy with more mental clarity, better concentration and less physical stress.

Sheila
Kauai, Hawaii

Thumb Healed

After smashing my thumb in a trailer hitch, Reiki energy stopped the bleeding and prevented bruising. For the next, approximately four days, I applied Reiki to my thumb and did not lose my fingernail. There was no pain even when squeezing the thumb. I forgot the injury was there.

Leonard
Kauai, Hawaii

New Energy and Clarity

We are home now from Kauai not quite a full week. Transitioning after our Reiki initiations has had its challenges but we seem to be coming through and I feel a real blossoming taking place. Reiki has been awesome for us. Speaking for myself, I have energy (I usually fell asleep 9:30ish, now I can stay up to midnight). With the new energy came clarity and focus and discipline which comes easily and naturally, I don't have to work at it. These are all things that were needed in my life. Morri and I will be setting up a Reiki practice here in Denver.

Alexis and Morri
Denver, Colorado

Flight Attendant Gives Reiki to Passenger

I am so thankful for my Reiki training. It was such a lovely and rewarding time. There have been a number of trying experiences over the past couple of weeks. Some were involved with my position as a flight attendant. There seemed to be more passengers needing a helping hand.

An old man was very ill on my last flight; he needed oxygen and was vomiting. I placed my hands on his shoulders for about ten minutes, which sent him to sleep.

After arriving in Los Angeles my friend who moved from Australia was having a hard time trying to make it in America. I gave her a full Reiki treatment to candlelight and the beautiful Reiki music. She was so happy, the next day she drove me all over L.A. and we parted both feeling much stronger and happier.

Nikki
Perth, Western Australia

Reiki Perks up Sisters-in-Law

Immediately upon completing my First Degree Reiki, I gave treatments to my two sisters-in-law. Josie was drained emotionally and physically taking care of my father-in-law for years with his stubbornness in changing his life and taking his medications. After 30 minutes of treatment you could see and feel the stress melt away. She was glowing with peace and contentment.

I was asked to give my sister-in-law Norma treatment. Her daughter and precious grandson who lived with her for two years were moving away to the mainland and she was sad and depressed. After 30 minutes of mini treatment, she was happy and talkative again. She also had that same glowing peaceful look.

Two weeks after my Reiki training, I did a fellow worker who had shoulder problems for years and took salmon oil every morning to deal with the pain. I treated him for 20 minutes and he felt better and no pain. I told him to thank Reiki and God, it's not me. The individual called me two weeks later and wants to take Reiki training. Reason being, he is pain free and wants to be a part of Reiki.

Russell
Kauai, Hawaii

Muscular Dystrophy Healing and Self-confidence Boost

My friend Lillian told me about Reiki, The Usui System of Natural Healing. I couldn't believe it was possible. My family has a history of Muscular Dystrophy and I was diagnosed with it myself.

There was constant discomfort in my left shoulder for over three years. And, I had a painful pinched nerve in my left foot causing me to use padding in my shoes. On the second day of my Reiki class, when we shared treatments with each other, my shoulder pain disappeared and has not returned. A few months later, after twice a day self-treatments, the pain in my foot was gone and predicted surgery was on longer needed. Another added benefit after Reiki was the ability to cut back and eliminate some of my daily medication.

The Reiki has also assisted me with more self confidence. I now enjoy participating in groups and sharing Reiki stories with others.

Jose
Kauai, Hawaii

Wrist Healing and Help for New Business

In doing stock work, in my shoe store business on the Big Island, I injured both wrists and needed to wear wrist braces on both wrists. I was not able to lift with either hand. This was a cumulative injury over eight years. After moving to Kauai, being initiated into Reiki and administering self-treatments, I no longer needed the wrist braces.

My sister and I wanted to open a cafe and bookstore on

Kauai. We were told it took months to get approval from the Planning Department. We put our business plans under the Reiki table during Reiki gatherings where they absorbed the positive flow of energy. Self-treatments assisted us to be centered and have clarity in our dealings. The results were that we interacted well with the Planning staff and the plans went through in ten weeks. After my daughters saw the positive results of Reiki, they received their Reiki training.

Joanna
Kauai, Hawaii

Freed of Pain...Dedicates His Life to Reiki

I was found by Reiki when I was searching for a way to relieve the pain caused by an auto accident 25 years ago. Reiki was supposed to help me through the surgery. That was in 1992. Reiki did more than that. It stopped the back pain immediately during the First Degree initiation. I canceled the surgery and I am now a Reiki Master and have dedicated my life to Reiki.

Carroll
Wolfeboro, New Hampshire

Reiki'ed Self to Wellness

After taking my First Degree Reiki training those 21 days of cleansing were intense. I felt like the floor had fallen from beneath me and I had nothing to hold on to but I held on anyway. Life has continued to get better and more wonderful since then. I talked my doctor into supervising my withdrawal from all medication including the Dilantin for seizures. I have Reiki'ed myself to wellness. I am so grateful.

Mary
Clementon, New York

Asthma Healed

For five years I had been troubled by a tight congestion in my chest along with a great deal of coughing and asthmatic wheezing. After three months of Shalandra's Reiki treatments I no longer have the problem.

Ed
Kauai, Hawaii

Allergies Healed and All Aspects of Life Lightened

Nine months ago I took my First Degree Reiki training, three months later I completed the Second Degree class.

Physical Changes:

My asthma and allergies are improving. I was taking inhalers and pills daily for asthma, a life long ailment for me. I'm now taking the inhalers occasionally and have had periods of time where I had no breathing troubles.

My allergies are markedly decreased. I'm taking less allergy medicine.

I have always been allergic to cats. I would not be able to even go to someone's house if they had cats. I have moved into my sister's house, she has many cats. Although they live outside, they are always around when I go outside. I am able to pet and play with them now without any allergy symptoms. I had never "felt" a cat purr before Reiki and now I am able to do that. I very much enjoy their company and companionship. Another allergy symptom that has disappeared is my eczema. I would have to put cortisone cream on the inside of my elbows, my face, and my neck. Now that has all cleared up.

I notice that I heal quickly. Before First Degree Reiki, I would take a week or 10 days to heal a cut. Now they heal in 2 or 3 days.

I'm eating healthier foods, less fat, less meat, more fruits and vegetables.

I'm exercising more.

My blood pressure was elevated because of stress in my life. Now it is normal.

I haven't had the usual winter colds and flu. In fact I haven't been sick all winter.

Emotional and Spiritual Changes:

A little over one year ago, my beloved husband died. He was in an accident and died suddenly and totally unexpectedly. This was quite a traumatic event in my life. Needless to say I had many, countless emotional issues to deal with. About nine months later I encountered Reiki. This is the area I have seen the most progress. The Reiki has helped me to see things more clearly and accept life's twists and turns. Many times having the Reiki energy has guided me through the grieving and depression processes that I have learned I must go through. I believe that I am able to move quickly and completely through the difficult steps because I have the Reiki helping me. It is truly a "God force," a loving energy, a guiding light.

Since the Reiki, I have had many growth opportunities. The cats have shown me that I still have a caring heart and that I can feel joy and contentment. The way was opened for me to get started in my beading work, something I've wanted to do for a long time. Just having the Reiki presence in our home has brightened and guided my children in their lives as they deal with the many teenage issues they have.

Currently, I am experiencing more clarity and connectedness with the world. I seem to understand nature things and people relationships at a different level than before. I seem to be more connected with the spiritual world, although I can see that I have lots to learn. I've made it through "my dark night of soul" and am starting to rebuild my life. I'm becoming more aware and able to contribute to life. Thank you Reiki!!!

Lei Lani
Kauai, Hawaii

Arm Heals . . . No Cast Necessary

Dan's daughter broke her arm on Thursday. The doctor wanted to cast it on Saturday. Between Thursday and Saturday, Dan and I did Reiki about 4 hours each day. On Saturday when it was supposed to be cast the X-RAY showed 2 weeks worth of healing and no cast was needed.

Sue
Crestone, Colorado

Successful Surgery and Relaxing More

I arrived in Seattle Tuesday night and gave mom her first full body Reiki treatment the following day. She was defensive but allowed me to do this. I continued to give her full body Reiki treatments every other day. Her second treatment came on Friday and she lightened up which made it easier for me. Sunday, before her third treatment, she brought up emotional issues that had been bothering her since childhood. I was so glad to hear these things surfacing, knowing that the healing process was in effect.

I proceeded with Reiki and she seemed more relaxed, probably because she knew what to expect. It appeared she was experiencing and taking notice of the benefits of Reiki. Monday, about five hours before her eye surgery. I gave her a short treatment. I kept a record of the things I felt in my hands during the sessions. There was definite healing progress in the body.

She has the beginning stages of emphysema so her breathing is a problem. I have been totally amazed every time my hands have been on her lungs, as her breathing changes and stabilizes, relaxing the body totally. At this time I feel she believes in the Reiki. Thank God for Reiki! Wait! That's not all.

Her surgery went so well and she started out so scared.

She never felt a stitch of pain and the symptoms that the doctors said she would probably have afterwards never arrived. During surgery when she realized that she was starting to stress, she made a conscious effort to relax. She learned the difference during Reiki treatments. I am so amazed! Every treatment besides the first one, her body went into total relaxation. I believe it helped her in surgery tremendously. The day after her surgery I gave her a short treatment on her eye. I did not feel the intense energy there I had felt before which tells me her body had adjusted well after the surgery. And, a day or so later mom asked me if I would give her more Reiki. Can you believe it? Now I'm talking to her about getting initiated into First Degree Reiki.

Amber
Anchorage, Alaska

Dancing with Reiki

For more than twenty years I have taught ballroom dancing on Kauai and have enjoyed my health, energy and stamina for teaching, performing and choreographing. When faced with challenges I relied on my faith in Christian Science and benefited from natural healings.

About two years ago I was scheduled for a six week course to teach a large, enthusiastic group of 40 adults how to dance the Swing. It is a dance which has many arm movements, some overhead or around the neck for turns. Swing requires balance for its many turns and quick footwork coordinated with both partners' quick arm movements danced precisely to the beat. And there are also arm movements blending into choreographed poses.

The day before this important event, I experienced much pain on my right arm and could barely lift it at waist level. It continued to hurt through the day and I had to keep it immobilized next to my body. That evening I was teaching a smaller class and just focused on the music, but as soon as I moved the arm, the pain was overwhelming and I found my attention divided between the pain and the class. Shalandra was present and provided a short Reiki treatment that helped to allow me to teach. I set an appointment with Shalandra for the next day. On my way to the dance class, I stopped to receive Reiki and even though I only had time for a half an hour treatment, the pain in my arm disappeared and has never returned.

During the Reiki treatment I was also able to discover the emotional reason for the pain. That benefit was an unexpected insight! I am very grateful for the divine energy that works through us to heal. Since completing the Reiki courses I have used this wonderful skill to assist in many situations for my family, others, and myself.

Alena
Kauai, Hawaii

A Reiki Master's Healing Story

It's the fourth anniversary of my diagnosis with breast cancer. Now I am approaching the fifth. With the aggressive type of cancer I have I should have been dead long ago! Instead, I continue to work on my own healing and am now involved with a most amazing group of people who are putting together an integrative medical practice. I work very well with them as I draw on my experience of being a patient and meeting so many different Reiki practitioners over the past four years. I know what it's like to face the medical establishment with an alternative perspective.

I declined the recommended medical treatments. I have not had the usual surgery associated with breast cancer. With the first round of cancer, I managed to avoid established medical treatment entirely. When a lump appeared two years later, I began to explore ways to work with medical treatment.

Right now, I am in complete remission. The past year has been a very difficult one in terms of the physical body and a very wonderful one in terms of relationship and healing. Reiki was an everyday experience for me for many months.

Two experiences were the most impressive. First, my partner and I would Reiki the cancer drugs before they were administered and then he would give me the complete Reiki treatment during the IV. He wants to start a program to initiate the chemotherapy lab support people into Reiki. My Portland, OR oncologist is a First Degree Reiki student and he was very supportive.

Reiki has been central to my being for the past twenty years. Reiki as a physical laying on of hands, by itself, did not heal me. Reiki, the Universal Life Force-God Power as Mrs. Takata called it-did heal me by guiding me to all the avenues needed to clear my body, mind, and spirit of cancer-making energy. The laying on of hands often facilitated access to my spiritual knowing and intuition about what I needed to do, work on, and visualize.

I have used macrobiotic eating, exercise, love, chemotherapy, bioenergetics, Rife, acupuncture, homeopathy, flower essences, past life work, anger release work, counseling and more to get to all that I needed. They have all nourished my new being-ness, along with Reiki. I do not know if it would have worked without any one part.

I'm grateful that I am stronger and wiser and more well each day. I'm going forward in life, trusting the process. I am being taught about the oneness of the universe and all its parts and how to find a true place of peaceful joy within.

A Reiki Master's story
Reiki Magazine International

Emotional Healing

Shalandra, your series of four Reiki treatments was excellent resulting in less stress. There were some powerful emotions that came up for healing. Now anger and other situations seem less of a problem. They were difficult circumstances and I seemed to handle them differently in a more positive manner. I recognized the patterns of what was happening, and with time didn't get angry, because I could see my mirror image of how I used to act.

The left side of the head, neck and shoulder still seems to bother me occasionally. I am more focused and things are flowing better. Situations are falling into place better and when they don't, I understand that its time to slow down. I see the messages better and know what I need to do. I realize now how important daily self-treatments are and that it isn't enough to do only half of the positions. They keep me in tune and flowing better with the energy of life. With the big mountains of personal garbage released, it is now easier to handle what is remaining for my complete healing.

A Reiki Student
Kauai, Hawaii

Burns Heal Miraculously

I was camping in Kalalau Valley on the Napali coast with some friends when I severely burned myself. In the dark of the night I reached down to move my friend's lantern and was unaware that it did not have a handle or a protective top on it. I ended up sizzling four of my fingers. One person commented that they could actually hear it.

We were out of ice at the time so I had nothing to cool it down with. I began applying Reiki immediately. I was in agony for a while but after a half hour or so the pain began to lessen and the burns began to blister.

We had kayaked to the valley and were leaving in a few

days. I was afraid that my hand would be too damaged and that it would be too painful to paddle home. To my relief by the time I went to bed that night the pain was gone. When I woke up the next morning, my hand was completely healed with just small scabs to show for it. Reiki got me home safe & sound!

Aimee
Kauai, Hawaii

Surgery Patient Revived and Tendinitis Healed

My friend's dad had surgery on July 29 in Colorado. After his surgery the medication made him disoriented. He did not know where he was, his conversation was not coherent, he did not realize that he had surgery and was not an ideal patient. He pulled his catheter out several times.

On August 2, his condition had not improved. He was on IV with nothing to eat or drink. I sent distant Reiki to him after lunch Hawaii time, and that afternoon Colorado time, he was allowed to have some Jell-O, ice tea and bouillon.

The morning of August 3, his doctor was amazed at his physical condition and his spirit. His doctor said it was a "miracle." He got to eat that day and, on August 4, he was released and went home.

After receiving my First Degree Reiki training from Shalandra, I gave my friend a half hour mini-treatment. The next morning, he told me that for years he had ringing in his ears. He went to a couple of doctors and the answer was always the same, "there is nothing we can do. You just have to live with it." The ringing in his ears had stopped after receiving Reiki.

Dini
Kauai, Hawaii

Asthma Healed

Shalandra, I can never thank you enough for all your help with my asthma. That Reiki is phenomenal! I have improved at least 80% overall, some days I go down a little and some days I am as high as 100%, not too many 100's yet.

I was so bad that I could hardly walk 50 feet. I just couldn't breathe. I was sure that I was going to die and was trying to put my affairs in order-but that's hard to do when you don't have the energy to think or make decisions. After almost two years of this you get pretty down in the dumps.

Anyway, thank you more than I can tell you!

Katie
Grand Junction, Colorado

Pain Gone

A 43-year-old man who injured himself by doing a flip from an exercise bar and fell with his head against his chest came to me for help. He had been hurting for 3 weeks and was on percodan medication and couldn't function without it. He had been on leave without pay and desperately wanted to get back to work. Treated him for two days and after the second day he stopped taking percodan and felt great. He went back to work the following week. He couldn't thank me enough for helping him with Reiki.

Puanani
Kauai, Hawaii

Self-Treatments Work Wonders

After receiving Shalandra's First Degree in April, I immediately could feel a change in my physical and mental being. Self-Reiki treatments, done both morning and night, enriched me with more energy and self-perseverance. I was able to complete a full day at work, standing 8 hours without pain, in my feet or back. Relieved by this, I noticed that I focused more clearly on sales and accomplished my monthly objectives.

One day in the kitchen I accidentally cut my finger with a knife. Immediately after I washed the blood away, I held my finger with my other hand for about 5 minutes. When I took my hand away, the cut was completely healed - I couldn't even feel which finger it was because the pain was gone also.

Luana
Kauai, Hawaii

Knee Renewed

My nephew who is away at college in Oregon and I were chatting on the Internet. He learned that I had the capability of sending a Reiki treatment.

During the conversation he mentioned that he hurt his knee while playing football. I asked him if he wanted me to send him a treatment and he said, yes.

The next morning, on his way to class, he found himself running up the stairs with no pain to his knee. He was amazed. He is no longer a skeptic to the Reiki energy.

Dini
Kauai, Hawaii

Female Organs Healed

While I was living on Vancouver Island, I had a miscarriage and as a result I had to have larpiscopic surgery through the belly button. My stitches popped the night I returned from my 4-day E.R. room nightmare. I taped my navel back together with surgical tape I had on hand. I went back to the hospital the next morning. The doctor said I did a good job and I was on my way to the healing process. Well, the pain in my abdominal muscles was so great that I decided to contact the massage therapist I had been using. I read some of her Reiki books waiting for an appointment and was aware of her interest in Reiki Natural Healing.

Wendy told me to come over and she would work on me. I am skeptical of everything but at the same time willing to try anything. At first I had a hard time clearing my mind considering the ordeal I had just been through. I could feel intense heat and energy coming through her as she was working on my head. As the healing energy transferred down toward my abdomen, I could feel a surge of energy go across my chest down through my abdomen and toward the area in my uterus and abdomen.

When I left, she said I would feel tired but then the healing would begin. I went to her 2 days after the surgery and from the moment I left her I began to heal. It was incredible so I have tried to spread Reiki information to other skeptics like myself.

When I went through the surgery, the Doctor in E.R. said he wanted to remove my tubes so that this would not happen again. I refused his decision knowing I might have to go through this painful operation again.

November 13 I have surgery scheduled in Michigan by a referred surgeon who said I have a blocked tube and he is going back in this time with a camera and a laser to clear the blockage.

I only went to Wendy for one treatment. I guess I felt so much better that I didn't go back. The burning sensation with a three-inch diameter around the navel seemed to disappear.

I came across your website and may be interested in taking some courses. I hope my story can be an inspiration to other women who are in need of healing.

Heather
British Columbia, Canada

Abnormal Cell Gone

In early September after a routine pap smear I was informed that my test showed abnormal cells in my cervix. I have continued to receive pap smears every three months since, receiving the same conformation each time.

After applying self Reiki, receiving Reiki from my partner, and monitoring my thoughts over the last few months, this last month's test has returned negative--I feel better than ever. Thank you for teaching us Reiki!

R.C.R.
North Carolina

Amazing Wellness Found

I am so happy, so excited and so thankful for Reiki. Here are some highlights of the first twelve-days of self-treatment. During and after class there was soreness in the abdominal area, cramps and diarrhea. The internal organs felt as if they had been moved or rearranged.

Day four, a popping sound in right ear was repeated 2 or 3 times, might I one day throw away my hearing aids? Day seven, Even though I was wearing my hearing aids I was having trouble hearing. I turned on the TV and took out my hearing aids to check the batteries. They were okay, but the moment I removed the hearing aids I had to grab the remote to turndown the sound. I was so thrilled but couldn't quite believe it. I no longer need my hearing aids!

Day five, at 4:00 a.m., I woke up with a headache and decided to do my self-treatment. Afterwards, I was feeling completely relaxed and was surprised to realize my headache was gone and I was not even aware of when it stopped.

Day five, my throat felt sore, the left tonsil was painful when swallowing. In working with the Reiki energy, I noticed a distinct difference between what I was feeling in my left and my right hand. Shalandra, I'm glad you made the statement several time in class to, pay attention to what you are feeling in your hands. I attributed the sore tonsil to sinus drainage that I attributed to a release by the Reiki energy.

Day six, my back was hurting from raking leaves. I rested on my lounge chair and placed my hands over the lower abdominal area, and in a few minutes the pain was gone and I felt so rested and energized, I went back to raking leaves.

Day seven, I'm no longer having trouble sleeping. I'm averaging 8 hours sleep per night. In reading the Reiki book from class, Reiki Energy Medicine, it mentioned something I had not even connected with Reiki. I've gotten in the habit of sleeping in a pair of warm wooly socks because my feet were always cold at night. In the past few nights I've had to remove them a few times because my feet were so warm they were perspiring.

Reiki is amazing. I'm so grateful that you come to Hot Springs Village to teach Reiki Natural Healing and I'm looking forward to taking my Second Degree training upon your return in April.

Lora
Hot Springs Village, Arkansas

Note: The above story was from a student's Reiki log book. Often, Reiki's many healing results are subtle. I usually suggest in class that students keep a log and notate these delicate results in order to understand more fully how each healing creates the results needed for the next priority. Once we understand how each healing was necessary before lasting results could be accomplished, we are usually in a state of total amazement regarding Reiki's complete healing process. ~S.A.

Shoulder Healed. He Couldn't Believe It Was True

Charlie was having trouble with his shoulder hurting and popping when he moved it. It was Saturday when I gave the Reiki treatment. I didn't hear from him Sunday. He called Monday morning to say, "I should have called you yesterday but waited until today just to be sure it was really for real that my shoulder was healed."

When I worked on his shoulder, I didn't need to feel the energy; I could actually see the muscles moving. What a joy it is to share Reiki with another person!

Lora
Hot Springs Village, Arkansas

Shingles Healed Overnight

On December 22 I had a severe outbreak of shingles. They were so painful, I felt like jumping out of my window headfirst. I had terrible red rash and blisters all over the left side of my torso and under my left arm. It was one of the worse outbreaks I have ever had.

On Christmas Eve I spoke with my friend Yvonne who had recently completed her First Degree Reiki training with Shalandra Abbey. She decided to come over and give me a treatment. While she was working on me, my left side was burning and tingling so bad. She finished the treatment and went home and I spent some time with my kids and husband and went to bed, waiting for Santa to arrive of course.

I slept through the night without any pain medication. When I woke up the burning was gone. I looked in the mirror at my body and I went into shock!!! I called my husband into the room and showed him my body where the shingles had been. The rash was completely gone, the blisters had dried up and I had already scabbed, that is a process that normally takes my body 2 weeks to happen! With Reiki Natural Healing it had happened over night!!! My husband and I were in complete shock!! I was so grateful I started to cry my eyes out. I had energy and my body looked 95% better than the day before.

Yvonne called and my husband, who is not a believer in anything other than traditional medicines, said to Yvonne, what is in your hands, what did you do to her, she is well. There is something magic in your hands. I was semi skeptical before and now I am a believer!!! Wow, I'm signing up for the next Reiki class...

Tammi
Kauai, Hawaii

Toxic Effects of Chemotherapy Lessened

Bradley was 11 years old when he was diagnosed with leukemia. He underwent chemotherapy for almost 4 years. The first month of chemo was intense. They had to kill the good cells as well as the cancer cells and so his immune system was actually down to zero.

He was admitted to Kapi'olani Hospital and 2-3 days later, they put a central line in his chest. He received injections once a week in his thigh with minimal side effects but treatment also involved scheduled 3-day stays in the hospital where chemo was administered directly into the central line. He always suffered intense headaches from these treatments. In addition, he had to receive regularly scheduled spinals, where the chemo was injected directly into the spine since the other treatments didn't reach this area. (Nature's way of protecting the cerebral system.)

With each spinal, anesthesia was administered until the spinal procedure was completed and Brad would slowly wake. These procedures made him so miserable and nauseous, he couldn't even sit up. The side effects from the chemo were extremely bad headaches, nausea, low back pain, and severe joint pain. In addition he had to deal with feelings of frustration and anger.

As his mother, I looked for things I could do to help him with his illness and his comfort. About halfway through this ordeal, I introduced naturopathic care and Reiki Natural Healing. I took First Degree Reiki training and started treating Bradley daily or whenever possible.

The first time I administered Reiki during a spinal treatment, I began while he was still asleep. He awoke and (miraculously) was about to sit up – and had no nausea! This was the outcome of Reiki for all the following spinal treatments.

With all the various drugs that Bradley received, although necessary, they were so toxic at times that neither Reiki nor naturopathic remedies were able to eliminate all the pain and discomfort. However, I believe Reiki did help Brad through his treatment and even more importantly, I believe Reiki played a part in lessening the buildup of residual toxic chemicals in his body.

Today, Bradley is 16 years old, healthy and in full remission, I am so glad I had Reiki to help!

Bradley's Mother
Oahu, Hawaii

Owns Responsibility for His Health

I've been an insulin "dependent" diabetic for 36 years. I've been a Reiki practitioner since 3/96. I received my Master training 6/99. Along with a low/no meat diet, insulin, Reiki and a conscious acknowledgement of my responsibility for being diabetic in the first place, I've been able to lead a happier, more productive life.

I don't get sick anymore and my resistance to disease is

great. My best suggestions are to own the responsibility for your health, which ties in with Reiki completely.

Kerry
Paxinos, Pennsylvania

Reading Glasses No Longer Needed

My entire family wears glasses; Mother, Sister, my Father wears tri-focals!! I have been giving myself Reiki self-treatment twice daily through both First and Second Degree training and have now rendered my reading glasses useless. These days I read more than ever and yet my eyes do not get tired and are not in need of correction.

Reiki has empowered me as a member of my family. I feel I can overcome these types of traits with the Reiki energy and ensure happier, healthier, generations to come.

Stefanie
Boulder, Colorado

Over-all Improvement in Fibromyalgia Patient

I am having great success with a fibromyalgia client. We have completed six Reiki sessions and although I thought she may take awhile she has started to really see improvements in her over-all life. It's just truly amazing to see her glow a little more each time she comes in.

Raina
Boone, North Carolina

A Way Out of Headaches with Reiki

When I was about 16 years of age, I started to develop deep, throbbing headaches. They continued on, often overpowering and at age 24 they found, with the newly invented CAT scan, that I had hydrocephalus. Water on the brain, as some refer to it. My brain produces about 12ccs of fluid per hour more than it reabsorbs.

The answer to this problem was simple - put in a shunting device to shunt the excess fluid away. But, theory does not always work and the headaches did not subside - even after 71 surgeries. Obviously, I turned to painkillers as a method of relief. It was not an appropriate means, but I think one can easily see the trap when they are on the outside looking in.

Think of the pain with no relief for the past three years except for a minor let up with drugs. Now add more drugs for more possible relief. It does not work. In fact, nothing I tried worked. Prayer, relaxation techniques, pain clinics, hypnosis, even distraction. No relief. Then, I met a Reiki Master named Shalandra Abbey who trained me in First Degree Reiki Natural Healing and offered me a way out of the headaches. I am now counting more and more days without headaches! This is my Reiki miracle that is happening with me!

Dave
Kauai, Hawaii

Pain of Migraines Controlled

I've never missed giving myself at least 2 self-treatments a day since my First Degree Reiki training. As far as my extreme headaches go they have been bad this year along with a complication of a bad back injury. However, with Reiki's assistance, I've been able to break the pain phases of the migraine within 24 hours every time, except for once. That is remarkable because there were times before my Reiki training it would take up to 3 full days. Yea for Reiki!!

Ginny
Littleton, Colorado

Old Pattern Gone

During my First Degree class with Shalandra, I noticed

myself looking at the floor a lot. My eyes weren't playing tricks on me – I perceived paisley-like patterns in the monotype carpeting. This visual perception had stayed with me from my years of experimentation with psychedelic substances. It was, quite actually, something I was accustomed to.

After the first Reiki initiation, the patterns disappeared and have not come back. Reiki has given me the strength to move past the psychedelic drug experiences and remain sober with the utmost grace and ease. My vision is now clear of these psychedelic patterns and Reiki Natural Healing has been the foundation of my journey to move through other patterns of behavior, thoughts, and ways of relating with everything in my life.

Anonymous
USA

Recovers from Fall

This story is about injuries I sustained about 14 weeks ago and how Reiki helped me recover. We had returned from an outing on our boat and had docked. I attempted to step from the boat onto our dock when my foot slipped and I started to fall into the water.

The water was still cold from the winter and I tried to lunge towards the dock and catch my fall by supporting myself with my arms on the dock. Of course, that did not work. Instead only one arm landed on the dock at an awkward angle. I dislocated my right shoulder, fell in the water after all and tore a hamstring in my left leg. I missed a rebar that was sticking out of the bottom of the lake by just a few inches.

The doctors told me that they felt I had also torn the rotator cuff, that I would more than likely have to have surgery and that I may not regain the full use of my arm/shoulder. They anticipated the hamstring repair to last 6 months to one year.

Well, the leg healed very fast, probably in 8 weeks. The shoulder is probably 90% recovered with no surgery, and improving all the time. I Reiki twice a day and know that I am blessed to be able to do so. I am looking forward to my Second Degree Reiki training when you return next summer.

Monika
Hot Springs Village, Arkansas

Goodbye Kidney Stones

One September morning, I experienced a severe pain on the lower left side of my back. I began to give myself a Reiki treatment but the pain intensified. I realized I had to get some help so started to go to Kalaheo clinic. On the way there, the pain became even more intense, so I drove directly to the hospital instead.

They proceeded to run a series of tests and I was diagnosed with kidney stones. The doctor gave me some painkillers and said he was confident that I could pass them.

When I arrived home the painkillers started to wear off and the piercing pain came back. This went on for a few days. My Reiki sister would call to see how I was doing and offered to come over and give me a hands-on treatment, but I was embarrassed to let her come over because I was in so much pain I hadn't done anything, not even showered in a few days.

She finally just came over and gave me a treatment. Afterwards the pain continued. My Reiki Master Shalandra Abbey and another Reiki Master Diane Ellis called on their way from the hospital to see how I was doing. When I told them I still had pain after the treatment they decided to stop by and check on me.

Shalandra instructed the Second Degree practitioner to work on my head area while the two masters worked on the kidney area. Immediately after they finished I felt 100% better and have been fine ever since.

I went back to the doctor for a check up, and although I felt no pain my doctor said I still had some signs of kidney stones, so she scheduled me for another sonogram and a few more tests. All the tests showed that I didn't have kidney stones.

Jeannine
Kauai, Hawaii

Sense of Smell Returns and Lowered Blood Pressure

Shalandra, after your Reiki introductory session, the first thing I noticed was that I could smell the individual fruit in the basket at home. I had been a 20 year smoker (I quit 10 years ago), and I had lost my sense of smell. Now this is a mixed blessing as I work in a nursing home. I'm only kidding. My new found sense of smell serves me well in all areas of my life.

The second blessing came when I decided not to have any major procedures done during the twenty-one day cleansing that occurs after First Degree Reiki training. I postponed my EGD. I had to go off my arthritis medicine for the procedure. After the procedure, I never resumed my arthritis medicine that I had been on for close to 10 years. I noticed the Reiki controls my arthritic pain so I can sleep when I go to bed at night.

Third, my arthritis medicine was the main culprit of my gastric reflux. The gastric reflux medication is very expensive and not covered by my insurance.

The fourth blessing came after I had been doing twice a

day self treatments for a while. It lowered my blood pressure and pulse. My doctor had to reduce my medication.

I have received other blessings I consider of a personal nature. In one month I recovered my cost for the course in decreased medical expenses. Plus, I got my Nursing credits!

An additional blessing comes from having found friends who also practice Reiki.

Nurse at Good Samaritan Health Care Center
Hot Springs Village, Arkansas

Cat Rebounds

My cat, Boots, who is now 24 YEARS OLD, was near death 3 years ago. He was loosing weight, his hair was falling out and his long black fur was turning brown! I asked my friend if she could give Boots some Reiki...which she did, two separate times for maybe 2 minutes each time. Boots would not stay on her lap any longer than that! Well, he gained 6 pounds, all his hair grew back in, nice and black and he started bounding around the house like a kitten!

Since I received your First Degree training I give him Reiki almost every day and he is still doing Great! Ahhh, the amazing power of Reiki Love!

HAPPY DAY!

Suzanna
Fort Lauderdale, Florida

Reiki Exchange Heals Lungs

It's been a challenging health year for me beginning with a mild heart attack in February, and then the discovery of three growths in my right lung. I decided not to have any invasive procedures beyond taking heart meds. Instead, I've done 80 exchange treatments with my Reiki students. The CAT scan last week showed that the cancer markers are gone in my lung. My artery is still plugged, so I'm going to keep up the sessions. It's been an exciting experience. I'm ready for a peaceful holiday season.

Gloria, Reiki Master
Oahu, Hawaii

Burn Healed

I was curling my straight-as-pins hair recently when the curling iron slipped from my hand and glanced off my right shoulder. Ouch! The burn was about the size of my thumb. I immediately broke off a piece of my aloe and smoothed the gel over the burn, put on a non-stick dressing and then I Reiki'ed it. It had been starting to "smart" painfully, but after the Reiki, there was no pain - AT ALL. My husband said perhaps I should put some Polysporin on it because it looked so bad. Well, I did and dabbed it off almost immediately because it started to burn. I reapplied some more aloe and continued periodically to Reiki it over the next few days. The spot healed completely within the week! Two weeks later there was only a very faint pale pink area where the burn had been. Yeah, Reiki!

Lottie
Hot Springs Village, Arkansas

Happy with Joy

I first took the class not knowing exactly what to expect. After many years of being not very happy (and even depressed at various times) I feel a real sense of well-being and even joy! I feel full of love and a gentle kindness toward others, very unlike anything I ever felt before. In addition after many years of chronic insomnia, I'm rolling over after my Reiki treatment and going right to sleep. Amazing!"

A Happy Student
Hot Springs Village, Arkansas

Pain Gone in Twisted Knee

Yesterday I went to an 80 yr old's birthday party in Waimea. A friend came with her Hawaiian boyfriend. I noticed as he came in that he was limping with a bandage around his left knee and he seemed to be in pain. After greeting him and the usual 5 or so minutes of small talk, I asked him what happened to his knee. He said that he fell and twisted it badly. When I asked him if he was in pain, he said, "Oh, not too much". I could tell that wasn't accurate but continued the conversation in another vein.

After about 5 more minutes, I looked him straight in the eye and asked him again if he was in pain, and he, this time, said "Yes, I am". I asked him to sit down at a table in the background, explained to him about Reiki and asked him if he wanted me to be the instrument to pass Reiki through me to him. He said "Yes, I would". We began with a prayer and then I went directly to his knee. For about the first 5 minutes I didn't feel much, and then all of a sudden it was just like a huge blockage was released, an immense amount of heat was felt and I noticed that he was in a very relaxed state as I continued for about another 25 minutes. As the flow abated I finished, and asked him to remain with his leg in the elevated position and got him a glass of water.

I took my leave of his presence at that time and went to chat with other party goers and get some food. After about 45 minutes he came up to me and said that the pain was entirely gone, he was walking up and down stairs in no pain and his leg and knee felt very light. I told him to pass on the energy to another in the form of an act of kindness, which he did within the next 1/2 hour when an elderly lady started choking on her food. He got her sorted out and I then told him privately that I noticed what he did and "good for him!"

Tom
Kauai, Hawaii

From Bedridden to Revived

On Wednesday March 23, I received a frantic email and then call from my daughter Carmel in Santa Barbara. It said that she received permission and needed to have Reiki sent to her friend Chris. He had been very sick for over a month and the doctors didn't know what was really wrong with him. She said, "I went to see him today and almost cried when I saw him. He's dropped 30 pounds and his bones are sticking out of his body like I've never seen. For the first time since he told me that he wasn't feeling well, I was afraid for him. He's on a liquid diet and can hardly keep anything down. He says at this point he's happy he's alive. I'm scared for him. I wish there was something I could do."

In her phone call she told me that he has been so weak that he can't even get out of bed, having been there for over a month now. The doctors thought it was some kind of intestinal bacteria, and he was given a drug, but the drug was making the problem worse. Another doctor took him off of that drug, but still couldn't figure out what was the cause. I called Hiroko, another of Shalandra's students, and she and I sent Reiki that night. I sent again at 4 am Thursday morning, again Thursday night, again early Friday morning at about 4:45 am, Friday night. This morning Carmel went to see him and called back astounded and amazed. He is not only up, but looking the best he's looked in a long time, eating, walked on a treadmill and walked down to the beach. He is eating yogurt as well. He is most grateful and asked Carmel to say thank you.

Tom
Kauai, Hawaii

Back Injury Clears Up

As I was getting ready to paint my living room I began to empty shelves of books and magazines and put them in boxes. Once the boxes were full I bent over and kind of tried to drag them. They must have been too heavy because I felt something snap on the right side of my back and then I couldn't stand up straight. I thought what the heck did I do now and would probably be laid up for a few days and couldn't start my painting.

So, I put heat on it and went into the hot tub that night and it didn't help, so and I had e-mailed Peg that night and asked her if she could send me Reiki that night.

I went to bed and could barely lie down because my back hurt, so I put a pillow under my back on that side which relieved the pain a little, enough for me to do my Reiki. As I proceeded to do my Reiki treatment, I got to the hip area and felt a release and all I could think was WOW!!! Did it really help my back and release the problem that easily? After I completed the Reiki self-treatment, I had to get out of bed to see if I could stand upright without pain and to my surprise YES!!! YES!!! The pain was completely gone! I learned a valuable lesson about what you told us in class to apply Reiki immediately to any situation.

Cindy
Hot Springs Village, Arkansas

Energy Cleared in New Home

We purchased a home in Kapaa which we remodeled with the intention of making it our new home. We were supposed to move in but I would feel uneasy and stressed about staying at our new place. There was a stressful energy and my husband and I would tend to bicker quite frequently at this location.

I called Shalandra so she could "heal" our home, and she did. She sent me the treatment report. That night, we slept at our old place in Kalaheo, better than ever, and when we woke up, we had this sense of closure, we were ready to move. I felt this energy, joy and enthusiasm to go to our new home. What a change! The energy felt peaceful, welcoming, loving, and nurturing.

Shalandra, thank you so much. My husband and I are having the time of our lives now. Much love, aloha and MAHALO!

Joanna
Kauai, Hawaii

Whales and Dolphins Too!

Someone once told me that whales don't sing when they are in their kitchen in Alaska but when they visit their bedroom in Hawaii and the Atlantic Ocean they sing the same story year after year, except each year they add another chapter to the story.

Soon after receiving this information I sent a distant Reiki treatment to the whales asking their permission to send and inquiring if they would like to exchange healing treatments. Receiving a positive response, I continued with their Reiki treatment which was an awesome experience in itself, but nothing compared to when I received my exchange treatment back from them.

That worked so well, I next connected with the dolphins and they too were wonderfully open to share energy healing treatments. It was exciting to notice how the overall energy of the whales was of a heavier, wiser nature than the dolphins. Theirs appeared lighter, more carefree and joyful! What Fun!

Shalandra Abbey
Maui, Hawaii

Dog Receives Healing in Four Legs

My dog received leg injuries so I administered Reiki. He

readjusted himself so that my hands were under his front legs, resting his paws on my arms. He stared straight into my eyes during the process and I swear I could feel Reiki energy coming from his "hands". It felt like we were both sharing the gift with one another. This morning, he's hardly even limping. One of the neatest experiences ever!!!!!!

Rhonda
Lamoni, Iowa

Ear – Pain Free and Hearing Restored

A big thank you to everyone who has been sending me Reiki to heal my ear!

Today, I am pain free and can hear again… I have been going around the house adjusting the volume down on the radio and TV. The chief surgeon successfully removed a solidified piece of ear wax the size of a kidney bean from my ear canal, despite using generic preparation, steroid suspensions and codeine, which made me far worse, my body could not tolerate any of these medicines, what did the trick was Reiki, olive oil and a warm water flush. Once again a big thank you!

Nessa
Kauai, Hawaii

No Sign of a Fracture

Do you know Shalandra, that the evening you put Don's name in your Reiki healing circle which would be the early hours of his night-time sleeping...he awoke and said, "Pam, I'm healed."

We didn't put the timing together until later! He'd been in your circle and was so ready to be healed!

He was scheduled for an MRI the next day and went ahead with it and they found NOTHING--although the orthopedic surgeon was convinced he had a stress fracture.

He's experienced some residual soreness here and there, but the crutches were gone and it's so wonderful!

We both thank you so much for including him in the Reiki healing circle. We would love to meet you!

Blessings and great thanks,

Don and Pam
Bristol, Tennessee

Circle Healing and Hands–on Treatment Revives Dad

I want to thank you very much for putting my father in your Reiki circle of Love and Light. I arrived in Miami on Sunday, went to see my dad at the Hospital and he was so weak, so skinny, almost could not speak. So, for about at least 2 hours, I just gave him Reiki. The next day they let him leave!!! They realized it was celiac, a syndrome that doctors can think is cancer or anemia but it is an intolerance to gluten, which blocks the intestines and digestive system inhibiting the absorption of food....He is doing GREAT!

Thank you so much.

Joanna
Kauai, Hawaii

Self Treatment Works!

Shalandra, Many Thanks for being my teacher. I really found the class to be just what I was asking the universe for...self healing and helping others and a possible career in my retirement in 10 years.

I do the self treatment faithfully cuz it is so beneficial to me energy wise. I have much more energy. Only one day I felt like I was so tired...but it is also that I am shedding a lot of toxic stuff that my body has been holding.

I plan to do the Second Degree training next year. My

niece actually is who inspired me to be open to Reiki. Her mom related how she helped heal with distant treatment her sisters' just adopted newborn twins. So when I saw the article in the paper about you offering a class; it was a clear sign to me.

I gave my second mini treatment to my girlfriend who had a bad cold and it was definitely a success. She could finally (after 5 days) breathe deeply as I laid my hands on her shoulders. And at the same time it gave me a boost of needed energy.

Elaine
Maui. Hawaii

Reiki Tunes Up Orchestra

Shalandra, I am enjoying my Reiki self-treatments and sending distant treatments to my family. I think I benefited enormously from taking Second Degree Reiki. I had a "strange" experience the other day. I was at an outdoor memorial service. It turned out to be a cold and windy day. I was ushering for my Rotary Club as volunteer service to the event and couldn't just leave. I also had not eaten supper so I was pretty miserable as this service (a concert) dragged on and on.

The music was horrible. It was so cold; none of the musicians could keep their instruments in tune. So the auditory expression was an assault on the senses as well. I started Reikiing myself so I wouldn't feel so miserable. Then I got this idea to send Reiki to the orchestra. To my amazement, within a few minutes they started to sound much better and played in tune for the rest of the evening.

Glenna
Minneapolis, Minnesota

Relaxation and Rejuvenation at Fair

I participated in the employee health fair at the Maui

Prince Hotel. It was the first experience for me to give Reiki treatments to "strangers" since earning my First Degree in Reiki from Shalandra Abbey a month earlier. I have been practicing Reiki on myself on a daily basis and had given "mini" treatments to a few friends and family members. The response had been favorable so I agreed to try offering it to people I did not know even though I was a novice.

I was pleased and surprised at the warm reception and acceptance of the people attending the fair. Not one person I treated had heard of Reiki but they were all very eager to "try it". Much to my relief, it was a very pleasant experience both for me and the "client". It was truly a positive and reaffirming experience for me to see their bodies relax and become rejuvenated as the Reiki energy passed through my hands.

I hope that through these "fairs" many more people will learn about the gentle healing that comes through Reiki treatments.

Elaine
Maui, Hawaii

Pre-birth Healing for Baby Chloe

Diane was pregnant with Baby Chloe when the doctors, after exhaustive testing, determined that, just like a previous child that the mother had, would die shortly after birth due to a very rare heart defect. They said that the ONLY thing that would save her would be a heart transplant at birth or a very rare heart surgery with an historically very low rate of success.

They were going to induce birth one week from when I was contacted. I began, along with Hiroko, another of Shalandra's students, sending Reiki morning and evening to Baby Chloe. Eight days later I was contacted with the news that Chloe was born and apparently healthy, but the doctors were due to come in the next morning to perform some intense testing to determine the state of her health.

Then I was called late the next evening to be told that she was in perfect health with nothing wrong with her heart. The doctors couldn't figure that out and said that they "MUST HAVE MIS-DIAGNOSED". They apparently didn't buy that Reiki and prayer had anything to do with the healing.

Tom
Kauai, Hawaii

Pain in the Neck Departs

I am a normal male of good health. I am 47 years old. Usually with a massage and a chiropractor treatment or two, I am put back into shape again to tackle the world. I had a recent incident where I had tightness in my left neck muscle around my collar.

This tightness was aggravating enough that the pain was severe to give me constant conscious pain. Being a pain that showed up all of a sudden, I thought it would go away after a day or two. It didn't. After a week and a half, I finally went to see a medical physician to get some idea of what might be happening to all of a sudden get this pain. I went into a massage therapist for neck massages for working the muscle. I tried heat packs, Tylenol, aspirin, hot soaked towels, and finally prescribed pain relievers (muscle relaxants).

I was getting exasperated for an answer. I had been putting up with the pain and constant tightness of the neck muscle, I continued seeing the medical physician and finally started seeing the chiropractor more. I was getting no relief.

At about the end of these six weeks of pain, I finally decided to see Amber, one of Shalandra's students, whom I know does the Reiki treatment. Now, remember, I had been dealing with this pain for 6 weeks, day after day, hour after hour. I was not afraid it was some weird disease but was getting to the point of needing relief from this pain and was wondering if I would find the right treatment.

My first moments of the Reiki treatment, I had total belief in the treatment that Amber would do. The treatment was non-invasive, non-threatening, and almost magical at the end of the hour treatment. After six weeks of constant pain, a doctor trying to give me a 'migraine' shot in my neck (I have NEVER had a migraine in my life), and several chiropractor visits, this one hour of treatment was miraculous. After one hour, my pain was gone. Poof! I am not by any means a sap or wimp. I walked away from that one hour of treatment completely free of pain. That pain did not come back the next day or the next week. It's been about two months. I am still without pain in my neck.

Fred
Anchorage, Alaska

Reiki Results in All-Over Goodness

Reiki has helped me in so many ways:

Physically:

1. "Frozen" right shoulder and arm- now 90% better

2. Pea-sized benign growth in throat-no longer can be found

3. Constant pain in lower right leg-almost gone

4. Pain in right side of neck and only 75% range of motion- now 95%

5. Back pain; easily hurt-only once in a great while

6. Minor aches and pains heal as soon as sufficient amount of Reiki applied

7. No colds; "allergy" recovery days have been reduced from 3 (w/meds) to 0 same day (w/o meds)

8. Eating more healthfully

Emotionally:

1. Much happier; not depressed

2. Not as angry, cynical, or sarcastic as I used to be

3. Not as bitter about men (and my relationships with them) as I have been known to be

4. More optimistic and hopeful like I was in my youth

5. Not as emotional and now able to be more objective, more often

6. Not as easily "hurt" or "wounded as I have been

7. More grounded, centered, balanced

8. More patient

Mentally:

1. Not as worried, nervous, anxious, harried, frantic, or borderline Obsessive/Compulsive as I used to be

2. Not as fearful or wary of being out in public or being in "social" situations

3. Not as forgetful; seem to remember more

4. Able to focus, concentrate better and more often

5. Thoughts are more calm; able to catch and release irrational thoughts much sooner

6. Helping to prioritize activities, errands, chores

Spiritually:

1. Closer connection, more often with God

2. Helping me to remember that I cannot do it alone and to ask for His help more often, and a lot sooner

3. Recognizing more easily, how often I am blessed, especially when He has given me the solutions to my problems

4. Helping me to be more trusting

5. Helping me to remember to be more grateful, more often

If I don't do Reiki at least twice a day I feel myself slipping back into my old "needs much improvement" self, and I have this feeling of emptiness. So, now I know that The more I do Reiki, the better I feel. I also feel better because I believe that Reiki is God's healing energy...

Ululani
Maui, Hawaii

Eats Better and No Alcohol

Shalandra, you can imagine how special it was for me to take your First Degree Reiki training. It's been a "Life Changing Experience" for me, Thank you. I already was a very positive person, but now, I'm sure about a lot more things.

I have practiced Reiki with people and could feel what was going on in their body...it was really something.

I'm doing Reiki twice a day on myself. I'm eating better and less. I've stopped drinking alcohol which is something I was trying to do for a long time. Thanks for everything.

Paulo
Bahia, Brazil

Headache Gone – No Charge for Taxi

My cab driver had a really bad headache and asked if I had an aspirin. I said no but that I could give him some Reiki Natural Healing. I think I only had time to do 3 minutes, but his splitting headache was so much better that he didn't charge me for the taxi ride because he was so grateful.

Linda
Gardena, California

Burn Healing

I recently completed First Degree Reiki training in Hot Springs Village, Arkansas. Shortly afterwards I returned home to remodel my guest bathroom. I burned my arm on the lights over the vanity as I was painting. I jumped off the vanity trying to decide what to do knowing it was a very bad burn. Remembering what you said Shalandra about treating burns in Reiki class I thought about my Reiki hands and the success stories shared. I covered the area and applied Reiki for only about 10 or 15 minutes and it never did blister. My husband asked me what happened, asked if I wanted him to take me to the doctor. I said no, that I was going to do Reiki on it. It hurt but I just continued. My husband said he didn't believe it, if he hadn't seen it with his own eyes. The burn was healed in 3 days. A miracle for sure!

Bea
Monroe, Louisiana

Reiki is Wonderful!

As a Second Degree practitioner I should be used to all the things Reiki can do, but still marvel when I hear and experience some of the wonderful happenings. It is hard to believe that I can actually be a part of such power and energy.

Since taking First Degree in April I have not even had one little cold and usually every year I have to take at least one round of antibiotics or more for an upper respiratory infection. It's WONDERFUL! My old shingles continue to be controlled by Reiki completely. You Shalandra and Reiki have been such a blessing in my life, thank you.

Joan
Hot Springs Village, Arkansas

Hospice Patient Calmed

Thank God for Reiki! I was called by Hospice yesterday to provide Reiki to a hospice patient in his "very soon to go" stage of life. It was beautiful, with the family all gathered and the amount of Aloha being shared. I did a bit of coaching, directing the two that were there helping him with the actual hands on physical needs towards areas drawing energy, while I worked on his neck, which was delicate as it was full of tumors.

What occurred was that the Reiki/God's Infinite and Unconditional Love was received and when we finished he had gone from a state of extreme body heat, fast breathing and thrashing about with pain to a state of calm breathing, a much cooled down body state and cessation of the thrashing. He was noticeably calm. More than anything, his loving family just showed so much aloha and respect for him. What a blessing and gift for me. I'm VERY grateful.

Tom
Kauai, Hawaii

Alzheimer's Patient's Agitation Relieved

Today two non-believers asked me if I would give Reiki to a very agitated Alzheimer's patient. I interrupted my lunch and put my hands on his shoulders for about 10 minutes. He drifted in and out of sleep. Then I asked him if he wanted to go lie down or go to eat. We assisted him to the dining room and they had no more trouble out of him for the rest of the day. I find that many Alzheimer's patients especially the advanced can't stand having your hands around their heads, but are very receptive to the shoulders. It doesn't take much time for them to calm down. I have started to begin a log of just work experiences.

Nurse at Good Samaritan Health Care Center
Hot Springs Village, Arkansas

Alzheimer's Patients Relax in Health Care Center

I have found that, in Hawaii, the elderly with Alzheimer's are quite receptive to laying hands on them, even on their head. When I do Reiki on them, I talk to them in a calm, soft voice while I have my hands on their head. Some crave loving, human skin contact and results are almost immediate. I can feel an enormous amount of energy passing through in a short period of time. So much so that my hands still tingle when I am done. I do not move to the eyes until I feel the body relax and trust has been established. Seems to work. And, yes, most of my "patients" drift into sleep after the treatment as well. What a Gift!

Nurse at Hale Makua Health Care Center
Maui, Hawaii

Breast Cyst Gone

I have a couple of Reiki miracle stories for you Shalandra. For the past 10 years or so I had a large cyst in my breast. At times it hurt a little. I was giving myself a self breast exam and discovered it was gone!!!! I was so shocked I kept checking to see if it was really gone and it was!!!! Thank you for your inspiration and support.

I just did a mini-treatment for a co-worker this morning. It was great, he had a severely pulled muscle in his back and his shoulder was very tense. What a world of difference the treatment made. Mahalo again!

Diane
Maui, Hawaii

Cancer Gone – Cries with Happiness

A family member in Bangkok was diagnosed with Cancer. They were going to give her medications to keep her comfortable for the next six months that is how long they gave her to live. I started sending Reiki every night and praying and recently I received a phone call from the husband of the family member and he said that they did some more tests on her and couldn't find the Cancer. It was gone! I was in tears because the family member was on the phone crying of happiness for about 30 minutes.

Lois
Hot Spring Village Arkansas

Migraines Relieved

A year ago I took your First Degree Reiki class in order to help my husband with chronic pain. It has lived up to my expectations in helping relieve pain, however what I did not realize was that while doing self treatments on myself I have eliminated my migraines. They just don't come any more. I used to have about one a week and usually had to take migraine medicine. Now they are gone and don't return unless I neglect my self treatments.

I work with a girl who is also plagued by migraines and she is interested in taking your class to see if it can help her. I would appreciate it if you could send the information on your next class in Hot Springs so I could pass it on to my friend.

Linda
Hot Springs, Arkansas

Third Degree Burns Healed in Ten Days

I use Reiki continuously, as much as I injure myself it's the only thing that has kept me alive. Last year I blew myself up - third degree burns that healed with no scars and the hair grew back. The fire chief said no one has ever lived through this kind of explosion. I used Reiki just afterwards in the ambulance and at the hospital, was told that my lungs should have collapsed; I should have had a concussion and brain damage. Reiki not only prevented this

- with many treatments the burns healed in 10 days. They told me they would take about 30 days to heal. And, you were right I keep looking younger, others opinions - not mine. Shalandra I continue to love life and its challenges and believing in the ability to heal, which are what you taught me. I was fortunate and grateful to have had you for two days alone in my private First Degree training.

Warren
Hendersonville, North Carolina

Doctor's Life Saved

I love to encourage others to receive Reiki treatments and training. The first Reiki story that comes to mind is about a 35 year old mother of three children who is a doctor in California. She was dying. Her husband runs their county medical system so they really believed in the medical system.

Three years ago she started losing weight, getting sick a lot, and had to quit her job. In August she was continuing to get weaker and confined to a wheel chair weighing only 90 lbs. During the three year period she had been to many, many doctors, receiving a variety of diagnoses. They gave up and sent her to the Mayo Clinic in the east for tests. After a week of tests she returned to California.

Two days later a call came from the clinic and informed her they could not find the problem and gave her 6 months to live at her rate of decline. Immediately Reiki treatments were started and it was discovered that chemicals were literally eating up her body. She found a health food store and started doing complete body flushes along with hours of Reiki Natural Healing.

She learned meditation and took massive doses of herbs to heal the tissues. In three months she stopped losing weight and in 6 months she had gained 10 lbs, and 9 months later was using a walker. Today this doctor is walking again, has regained her weight, and is back to work part time, and getting stronger with each passing day.

Warren
Hendersonville, North Carolina

Number One Closer Now

I have been in sales for a long time now. I am a sales executive for a highly competitive company. Feeling I needed energy, physical and mental, I called Shalandra for an appointment so she could send me Reiki's healing energy.

The result has been an extremely successful year. I went from middle of the road to number one closer. I had three months when my income was way over $30,000 per month.

After that I was not selling as much. I ordered more Reiki treatments again and I sold a TRIPLE Down. Three people bought from me in one day!

I am very grateful for the Reiki energy. It is marvelous and it is a great way to remember that sales is about energy, about exchanging and giving them your best, and the benefit of a great product that is going to bring love, joy and fun to THEIR lives.

Joanna
Kauai, Hawaii

Loan Accepted After Reiki Treatment

Reiki energy worked a miracle, I mean seriously! I am in the mortgage business. Recently I had clients, a hard working couple, who were buying their first home. The mortgage they were approved for was under a special program available for a limited time. If you can picture this, loan is approved, buyers are excited and we are waiting for the closing documents to arrive via email.

Then I got "the phone call". The loan had been audited
by the quality control department of my company and was
being turned down; the condo development was not
acceptable. The buyers would not be able to move into the
home and loan was unequivocally rejected. And there was
no other loan program that the buyers could qualify for with
the amount of money they had to put down.

I was between my First and Second Degree Reiki
training at this time and though I thought the case was
hopeless, I sent out a very distressed email to Shalandra and
ordered a distant Reiki treatment to clear the energy for
this impossible situation?

A few days passed and nothing much seemed to happen.
Then for some reason, my boss (who is always super busy)
decided to make it her "cause" to get this decision
overturned.

It is almost comical looking back on it, over the next
week more and more "mainland" managers in mortgage
financing got involved to the point where they were falling
over each other making suggestions and disagreeing on the
appropriate resolution which caused a 2 week delay in
getting an answer. Meanwhile my buyers are about to get
evicted from their rental (where they had given notice after
our loan approval). It was a real cliffhanger at this point!

Shalandra had cautioned me that the Reiki answer
would be for the highest good but I really was just worried
about my clients at this point. After about 3 weeks people
high up in my company (a huge corporation) had several
conversations with the lender (to whom they sell the loans
after they close) in Washington DC. Finally we got the
news. Not only were my buyers being approved, but going
forward, anyone wishing to buy a home or condo that was
offered by the lender under this program would not have to
worry about the property being turned down. The situation

was discussed and resolved on a national level with the largest purchaser of residential loans in the country. They buy closed loans in large batches and in my 28 years in the mortgage business I have never seen them look at the merits of an individual loan. This was huge.

So the loan closed, mission accomplished, and my clients are ecstatic. Plus the favorable Reiki resolution of this issue will benefit many future buyers.

Reiki energy healed what I thought was a lost cause. And now I have my Second Degree Reiki training completed and I am happy to say that I recently sent distance Reiki to my own housing situation as I could not find a place that suited my needs. Within a few days I found the perfect space, convenient and peaceful, that I will be moving into at the end of the month.

Thanks for letting me tell my story and thanks Shalandra for being a great Reiki Master.

JT Alexander
Kailua Kona, Hawaii

Dogs Healed After Being Hit By Car

I love our two Jack Russel dogs Tillie and Sadie; they are loyal and go with me everywhere. Tillie found her way into the street and was hit by a car. She was very weak and could hardly walk. It was clear that her spine was out of alignment and her back right leg was hurt badly. After several visits to the vet and much medication we were told that she would need to live with her spine out of alignment and probably limp for the rest of her life.

I am a Second Degree Reiki practitioner and was assisting her with Reiki during this time. After this diagnosis I called my Reiki Master Shalandra Abbey and ordered a series of four distant Reiki treatments. After her first treatment Tillie was much improved. Her appetite was

better and she was drinking more water. The most
noticeable deficit was in her walking, though all four limbs
seemed to work, they were not in unison and she would fall
over...I was concerned about her spine as it seemed to curve
like an 'S' with the rear pulled to the right side. It was
absolutely improved after the first treatment.

Following the second treatment she actually was
wagging her tail. Something I hadn't seen in awhile
probably due to the stiffness of her back.

The third treatment her spine looked completely
straight and the little hump in her back was totally gone.
She was so much improved. Tillie was actually able to go up
and down the backstairs of the lanai, which was amazing to
see because before she had to be carried. She wobbled a bit
going up and down but was definitely improving. She could
get on the couch by herself and walk around. It was an
unbelievable transformation to see. Her eye seemed to be
clearing up a lot more - the big gash above her eye had
receded. Also there was injury on the side of her face and it
seemed like a lot of the swelling had gone down. I was
thrilled to tears.

The fourth treatment Tilly cuddled up to me and put
her head on my heart. I continued to do hands on Reiki all
over her body and witness her ongoing healing. During this
time her sister Sadie would look worried and put her head
on my shoulder.

Tilly, our Jack Russel was on her way to better health
and healing. I think its remarkable how she is doing. I told
Shalandra that I love this little dog and to please feel free to
send her as many Reiki treatments as she needs to get her
well. She needed a series of four.

What followed this innocent is still hard to believe. The
following week Sadie went into the road and was hit by a

car. Again after Shalandra's first distant treatment Sadie
seemed much better. She slept through the night for the
first time since the accident. She had not had a bowel
movement until right after the second treatment. Sadie also
had an energetic release shortly after her second session
where her whole body started to shake and then subsided.
There appeared to be major healing taking place. What was
noticed most after the third session was a little more
shaking resulting in her holding her head up higher when
she walked. After the fourth session Sadie appeared to be
like a new dog just a little weak from the ordeal. This was a
horribly close call for our beloved beings I am sure they
could not have made it without Shalandra's Reiki support. I
guess we have Reiki dogs now!

Faye
Kauai, Hawaii

Dog with Cancer Benefits from Reiki

I love my Reiki Shalandra. It is such an important part
of my life. Our little dog has recently been diagnosed with
cancer and I have used Reiki on him. The vet is very
pleased with his blood work and I attribute it to Reiki.
Hope to see you in the spring.

Judy
Hot Springs, Arkansas

Newborn Calves Revived

In north Missouri the calving season of March and April
can be very cold and wet. When a heifer has her first calf
sometimes she doesn't know where the best place to give
birth will be. She chooses a ditch out of the wind, but in the
mud and water in the ditch makes it an awful place to come
into the world.

Baby calves get chilled very quickly. We have had

several calves born this year and we have brought them to the barn where I have been able to give them Reiki. One in particular was making a bubbly sound when it breathed. After the Reiki treatment the breathing was better and the little calf is now doing very well. Thank you Shalandra for my Reiki!

Lisa
Eagleville, Missouri

Reiki Heals Shoulder After Surgery Fails

I had rotator cuff surgery after an MRI showed that I had a completely severed supraspinatus tendon, which is the one that goes from the arm across the top of the shoulder. It allows you to raise your arm directly over your head, among other things.

The surgery, scheduled at the end of September, was difficult but we were all hopeful, and I was diligent about doing my physical therapy as prescribed. I knew it would be a long process, but as time went on I was beginning to get frustrated that I didn't seem to be improving.

So by December when I really wasn't making any progress in my strength and range of motion but I was continually in pain from constant inflammation in the shoulder and arm from my intense therapy, the doctor ordered another MRI to see what was going on inside my shoulder. The MRI revealed that due to the weak tissue in my shoulder, the tendon had not held and was not attached at all. The doctor showed my test results to every other orthopedic doctor in their group to get each doctor's opinion as to whether or not a second surgery should even be attempted. The overwhelming response was no. My only option at that point, from their perspective, was to continue physical therapy in an effort to strengthen every other muscle in my shoulder area, which includes the back and arm, to try and teach those muscles to in effect do the job that the severed tendon had done.

So I worked hard on the therapy. And I continued to have a lot of inflammation that not only was painful but restricted my progress. It seemed like a no-win situation.

Then in January I had my first Reiki treatment. It was incredible! All the pain from the inflammation was gone! This was wonderful! And then on my next visit to physical therapy they overworked my shoulder and all the pain was back again. So I started to rethink my treatment and options. I changed physical therapists. And by March, after my 3rd Reiki treatment I decided to study Reiki and completed my First Degree training with Shalandra so that I could continue to practice self-treatments to further my shoulder healing and rehabilitation. In less than a year I attained full use and full range of motion in my shoulder. And, miraculously, the general consensus from all trainers and massage therapists that I've worked with is that my supraspinatus tendon is attached and functioning properly!

Barbara
Denver, Colorado

Hearing Restored

I would just love to heal my eyes, but as Reiki Practitioners we know Reiki Natural Healing always goes the area most needed at the moment.

Mom was totally deaf in her right ear and almost totally deaf in the left when she passed. I had noticed my hearing was going out of the right ear about the time she left. I felt almost doomed to the same fate since there is a long family history of it. There is even a very old photo of my Great-grandmother with a megaphone to her ear. I guess in those days they thought that might help. Because my hearing was getting so poor in the right ear I just got in the habit of using the left ear for the telephone. For some reason the other day I couldn't use the left ear and I held the phone up to my right ear and low and behold I could hear just as well out of the right ear. When my hearing was restored beats me. I don't know if it was gradual or sudden onset. But I am willing to give the credit to Reiki because of all of it's healing energy I have been receiving.

Lesley Case RN, BSN, Reiki Master Candidate
www.ReikiArkansas.com
Hot Springs Village, Arkansas

She Loves Reiki and How It Heals and Transforms Lives

I love Reiki! It is helping me deal with a multitude of stresses at work and at home. My dog is healing incredibly well, and I am trading Reiki for all kinds of favors with family members. The trade off is well worth it. We all benefit.

I am doing Reiki self-treatments every morning and every evening as well as at least one mini or full treatment on someone else daily. I am very impressed with your teaching and can understand how Reiki has transformed yours as well as other's lives! You have such a kind, warm, loving spirit.

Judy
Long Beach, California

Reiki Heals and Brings Inner Peace

After so many childhood tragedies and disappointing events, I was in constant search of the right counseling, massage, workout, class, book after book, church, vitamin, relationship, whatever…to find inner peace and contentment. I felt like I finally "had" it when I was baptized for the 1st time. But that bliss and euphoric peace only lasted 5 days, and then my youngest son was in a tragic motorcycle accident (and even more horrific 2 month hospital stay) just 2 days after his 18th birthday. He was in a coma, had a traumatic brain injury and was unable to walk, talk or eat. He couldn't even push his call button if he needed help. He was full of hardware to fix his broken bones. I quit my paralegal job and brought him home to strive for his optimal health. I juiced fresh live food for him and kept his environment positive and cheerful.

I poured all I had into him but forgot all about taking care of myself (well, and honestly just didn't know how—he needed so much time and energy, and I was his sole caregiver.) He has made a "miraculous" recovery and I have no regrets!

However, at the end of those 2 years, I was so far away from "bliss" that I had no idea how to get it back. I had daily headaches that I curbed with Excedrin. I was exhausted to my core, melancholy, and extremely depressed. I found comfort in drinking but only for a couple hours—and felt worse in the morning. I was unmotivated to exercise and had gained weight to the point that my kids were disappointed in me (but I didn't care). I was terribly broken-hearted over what happened to my son (coupled with guilt for not being grateful for his miraculous progress). His accident seemed like a cruel joke in my life (icing on the cake so to speak) and I started to feel suicidal (although this is the 1st time I've admitted that).

Since my 1st of many visits to Maui since 1985, I have found it to be a healing and rejuvenating place—so I booked my ticket, fortunate enough to have a girlfriend there with an extra room for me. I did nothing but rest and sleep for about a week. I then found Johanna's flyer and called for a massage. But for some reason I told her how I was feeling and she graciously recommended Shalandra Abbey for Reiki. Huh?! What's THAT?! With John

Mellancamp song playing in my head for the past month about my energy going wrong, as well as a new friend telling me I needed "energy work"...I called her. Hearing my voice she recommended a series of 4 treatments, 4 days in a row. She was so right.

One treatment would NOT have done the work! However, after the 1st treatment, I wasn't so sure about going back. It brought up so many deep emotions that I felt like I couldn't breathe and my head may explode in a ball of fire. I sobbed. But I stayed—and went back for more! I slept through the other treatments, which were peaceful and relaxing. I also slept so well at night after these treatments—better than I remember EVER sleeping in my life before.

Shalandra recommended learning Reiki for self-treatments and also to work with my son when I got home. What a wonderful blessing and experience! I started self-treatments a few days ago and already I know my life is forever changed for the better. I feel so calm and peaceful. I woke up with a headache this morning and felt a head cold coming on (those planes!) but was able to Reiki through the headache and not grab Excedrin. In fact, I haven't had any since about day 2 of Shalandra's treatments.

A major source of the headaches came from an area in my neck that was constantly stiff/swollen and painful—but that is no longer swollen and only has minimal stiffness. I have no doubt that will completely clear up in time and further self- treatments. In addition, my eyes would burn and water off and on for the past few months, but that has completely cleared up. I feel inspired to walk, start yoga, and be my best. I have a new appetite...which doesn't want to indulge in things that may dull my new-found senses. I noticed today while driving that I feel like I have new eyes...colors and images are sharper, clearer. I am in awe of things...like seeing them for the 1st time. It's strange yet wonderful. I am moving much slower, more graceful is how

I feel. I also saw an old man in a wheelchair without legs whistling today. He struck me so deep and made me smile…the feeling of "all is right in the world" was in his whistle. And that is exactly how I feel.

My 1st "client" was our dog, Sadie, who was hit by a car recently and hurt her leg. She was moving around okay when I got home but I did the treatments on her anyway. I could feel the heat in her injured leg. She seemed like she was in a trance and now follows me everywhere wanting more! I also did a mini-treatment on my middle son who fell asleep sitting up by position 4!

I will be returning to Maui for Second Degree Training with Shalandra. I feel so blessed with this gift that I want to share it with others and also continue on this peaceful path. Shalandra is inspiring!

Rhonda
Bellingham, Washington

Reiki for Infected Wound

Nancy gave me Reiki three 3 or 4 times for a big wound on my leg. The doctor thought he would have to send me to the wound clinic but gave me a week to decide. When I came back he was away but the nurse practitioner he had chosen to make the decision put a needle in to draw out some of the infection but got nothing and said she was surprised as she had seen the swelling and redness the week before.

I just soaked it in warm soapy water for an hour every day and gave it more Reiki. I feel very blessed.

Sally
Hot Springs Village, Arkansas

Distant Reiki Treatment Helps Emotional and Physical Symptoms

Hi Shalandra, thank you!! Your distant treatment was

incredible and removed emotional blockages that I had been holding onto during a particularly challenging situation that occurred 2 years ago in Maui.

I certainly wasn't aware of the impact this past experience had permeated my life until your treatment. It was immensely overwhelming emotionally, following the release I experienced no pain at all in either hip. Today was a little challenging regarding physical sensations, however I feel fantastic. Thank you, it was definitely a WOW!!"

Rev. Jennifer
Maui, Hawaii

Reiki Takes the Itch Out of Mosquito Bites

Monday night before our Reiki Circle, you may remember, I was bitten a few times by a mosquito (or 10). I have always been a magnet for them and as a child, during the summers, would be covered with scabs and scars from bites I couldn't stop itching. Monday night, as I was scratching away Lula said, "Why don't we try Reiki?" She placed her hand on my arm for a few minutes until the group was called together. In a few moments the itching was GONE and didn't come back. As I drove home that night I was thinking, "Why didn't the thought of doing Reiki on myself come to me a naturally as it had to Lula?" I don't expect that to be the case ever again. Normally, bites ebb and flow with me and days later I could still be having a reaction but not this time! I still have small welts but they aren't the angry red ones that I would have had before Reiki. I have yet to build the "mosquito bubble" around myself; it will come. In the meantime, I've been very successful with applying Reiki to myself to stop the itch.

I look forward to taking the Second Degree class with you.

Linda
Powhatan, Virginia

As you have learned from the information and examples in this book, Reiki is not only a complete healing modality that leads to better health, but can also become a "whole" way of living that flows with source energy and ultimately leads to personal freedom on a very deep level.

Reiki uplifts and engages our consciousness in soul, mind and body while bringing enhancement to the well being of situations and conditions, as well as to all life forms.

We can rise to a higher state of living by giving and receiving Reiki and connecting with the life-force energy of all things. The freedom that comes from this opens us to a new awareness as we enter a new era of spiritual understanding and evolution on planet Earth.

May you continue joyfully on your journey of unlimited possibilities!

INDEX

ABOUT THE AUTHOR

Shalandra Abbey discovered a simple way to heal herself and other people through Reiki in 1988. She left the IBM Corporation in Coral Gables, Florida in 1990 and moved to Kauai, Hawaii to live the life of a full-time Reiki Master. Since that time she has been a member of The Reiki Alliance—an international, professional organization of Reiki Masters.

Her classes are approved for continuing education credit by the Hawaii and Arkansas Nurses Association and the National Certification Board for Therapeutic Massage and Bodywork. She is a guest speaker for various organizations and has appeared on several radio and TV shows.

Shalandra provides hands-on and distant treatments and trainings in Hawaii, on the mainland and internationally. As she travels she is in contact with hospice, hospitals, clinics, business groups, churches, etc. to assist them in establishing Reiki programs in their areas. She currently resides on the island of Maui, Hawaii. Ms. Abbey can be reached through her website: www.ReikiHawaii.com

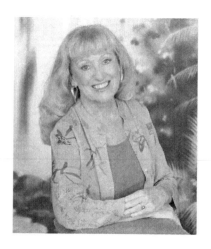

www.ReikiHawaii.com
for
Gift Certificates
Reiki Training Calendar
Reiki Treatments: Hands-on and Distant
Reiki Calendar of Events
Reiki Tables and Supplies
YouTube Reiki Introduction
Downloadable Study Guide for this Book
Plus More Valuable Reiki Information

Quantity Discounts Available for This Book

Ideal for
Reiki Masters who offer books in their classes
Healthcare organizations
Anyone who wishes to sell or give as gifts

Living a Life of Reiki is also available to
download as an eBook, and for
Kindle Reader and Nook
See details and order at
www.ReikiHawaii.com

REIKI CD FROM SHALANDRA ABBEY

Self Treatment for Reiki Practitioners

This CD was created for students of Usui Shiki Ryoho. The information on it supports what you have learned in class after receiving the sacred initiation to start the flow of Reiki energy.

After more than twenty years of practicing Reiki and teaching hundreds of students around the globe, Shalandra Abbey created this CD as an encouragement and reminder of the importance of self-treatment, the foundation of our practice.

It isn't always easy at first to get in the habit of daily self-treatments. At first we may simply forget about it and then later try to catch up. As the habit starts to feel pretty good, then better and better, we may realize we need less sleep, our schedule starts flowing with less effort throughout the day, and synchronicities often become commonplace. We start to feel a respect for ourselves on a new level, don't get sick as much and feel more alive then we could ever remember feeling before. We realize by then that we wouldn't dream of not doing self-treatment.

It has been the number one priority in my life for over twenty years and counting. If this CD encourages you to do more self-treatment and brings you greater health, love and harmony in your life, then I am satisfied that it was worth the effort it took to produce it.

Order at www.ReikiHawaii.com

Available in CD format or as an instant download
for i-Pods, computers or other mp3 players

**Quantity Discounts Available for
Reiki Masters to Offer in Classes or give as gifts to
students of Usui Shiki Ryoho**

Visit www.ReikiHawaii.com for
details and to listen to the first track

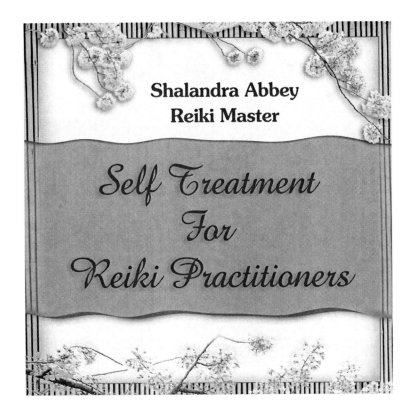

Shalandra Abbey
Reiki Master

*Self Treatment
For
Reiki Practitioners*

CPSIA information can be obtained
at www.ICGtesting.com
Printed in the USA
FSOW01n2151210415
6532FS